# The Midlife Male Handbook

## A Man's Guide To Thriving Through Andropause

**JAMES DAVIS**

**Synergy Publishing**
Newberry, FL 32669
publishwithsynergy.com

**The Midlife Male Handbook**
A Man's Guide To Thriving Through Andropause
By James Davis

Copyright© 2025 by James Davis

All Rights reserved. Under International Copyright Law, no part of this publication may be reproduced, stored, or transmitted by any means—electronic, mechanical, photographic (photocopy), recording, or otherwise—without written permission from the publisher and copyright holder.

Printed in the United Kingdom.
International Standard Book Number: ISBN 978-0-912106-39-7

Interior Layout and Cover Design:
Cris Convery

**Disclaimer:**
Before beginning any exercise programme, please consult with your physician or healthcare provider. The information provided by this book is intended for general guidance and educational purposes only. The exercises and activities outlined in this book may not be suitable for everyone. It is important to listen to your body, make modifications as needed, and stop any activity that causes discomfort or pain. By engaging in the exercises in this book, you acknowledge that you are doing so at your own risk. The author and publisher of this book are not responsible for any injuries or health issues that may result from following the exercises provided.

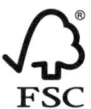

# CONTENTS

## Part 1: The Knowledge
4 Why We Need This Book
5 Introduction
13 About Me
16 Things You Probably Didn't Know But Should
18 The State We're In... All About Testosterone
26 Understanding Andropause And Its Impacts
28 Who Is This Book For?
31 Let's Talk About Those Big Midlife Challenges
36 Reality And Outcomes
39 If You Want, You Must
41 Here's What We Need To Be Doing
45 Your Performance Principles In Detail
45 Performance Principle 1: Life Equilibrium
47 Performance Principle 2: Understanding Hormones
50 Performance Principle 3: Nutrition
56 Performance Principle 4: Understanding And Managing Stress
61 Performance Principle 5: The Power Of Exercise
66 Performance Principle 6: Sleep And Recovery
67 Performance Principle 7: Transforming Habits
70 Performance Principle 8: Building A Positive Mindset
77 Performance Principle 9: Connection, Values, Passion And Purpose
82 Performance Principle 10: Supplements
84 Bonus Principle: Accountability
86 A Summary Of The Principles
88 Objections
100 Ask Yourself This

## Part 2: The 30-day Programme
106 Programme Introduction
108 Plan Summary
112 Setting And Committing To Goals
114 Mindset
116 Nutrition
130 Movement
143 Week 1: Life Equilibrium
148 Week 2: Vision Setting
154 Week 3: Habit Shift
158 Week 4: Future Self
161 Conclusion
162 A Final Word
164 Next Step
165 References

# Part 1
## The Knowledge

# Why We Need This Book

*Midlife can be challenging for both men and women, but let's look at the statistics.*

The single biggest killer of men up to age 50 is suicide. After 50 it's heart disease, yet males aged 50 to 54 have the highest suicide rate of all. In fact the suicide rate for men aged 50 to 54 is almost five times greater than the rate for women of all ages.

Men who commit suicide at midlife tend to have lower testosterone levels. Low testosterone is a risk factor for heart disease, and at midlife men can be starting to feel the effects of low testosterone more than at any other time in their life, which can bring a host of physical, emotional, mental and psychological symptoms. In a report on ageing, 48% of men in England experienced some degree of loneliness, with 14% experiencing moderate to high degrees of isolation. The main drivers for this are a lack of support systems, difficulties with emotional expression, retirement or redundancy, divorce and poor health.

*"The average 22 year old today has lower testosterone than the average 70 year old had just 50 years ago."*

On top of that testosterone levels are falling in the developed world.

The average 22 year old today has lower testosterone than the average 70 year old had just 50 years ago.

Testosterone is a vital hormone, assisting with a range of physical and psychological functions that have a positive effect on wellbeing. Yet testosterone is stigmatised. We need to start talking about it, undo the stigma, and start helping men not just survive, but thrive.

That is why we need this book.

# Introduction

*There it was. Yet another friend in his 40s telling me that this was it. That from here it was all downhill. That expanding waistlines, low energy, low libido and a general lack of get up and go, was all that was left. If I had to sum it up in one word? Apathetic. Apathetic about his life, his career, his relationship and his health.*

Does this sound familiar? Because I can tell you this isn't about one person, it's about 'midlife men' in general and it's more common than you'd believe.

As far as he was concerned this was the beginning of the end. It was time to stop moving forward and accept decline. To be honest it made me so frustrated. I was in Ibiza running health retreats, seeing hundreds of clients a summer, seeing the same issues arising, hearing the same views from those in midlife and you know what? It really distressed me.

At the time I was in my 40s and I wasn't feeling this way at all, nor were other guys that I hung out with. I'm in my 50s now and I still don't feel that way. You know why that is?

Because I understand what's going on with men's hormones in their 40s and beyond. I understand what I need to do to work with them, to get the best out of life, to feel energised every day, to still fit into the same jeans size I was in in my 20s, to still have a healthy libido, to want more from life.

So if you're feeling like you're not at your optimum in terms of performance levels, energy or you are struggling with your mood, don't worry. It's fixable. When you don't know or understand what's going on with you internally, you can't know how, not only your body, but your mind and emotions are being affected. Importantly, if you don't know what you are dealing with, then it is impossible to know what to do about it.

I'm here to tell you that there's another way. A way that means you don't have to make massive sacrifices in your life and give up the things you love like alcohol, and good food. That you don't need to be spending hours a week working out, but that you can feel energised, confident, positive, ready to carpe diem, every day.

Yes, you'll have to work for it, but wouldn't you rather do a little bit of work to feel great, as opposed to doing nothing and feeling terrible?

## CASE STUDY: **J (46)**

J came to me exhausted, burnt out from work, and barely connecting with his family. We worked on outcomes, what did he actually want?

Then we devised a plan of regular movement, cleaned up his diet and spent time on tools to help deepen communication, as well as looking at values and purpose.

After 30-days, his energy skyrocketed, he dropped inches from his waistline, but most importantly? He rediscovered his passion for life, started making time for the things and people that truly matter, and felt more alive than he had in years.

In his mid-40s, J was exhausted and on the verge of burning out from years of overworking.

His once-thriving career had taken its toll on both his physical and mental health. He found himself constantly fatigued, relying on caffeine just to get through the day. More worryingly, his connection with his family was deteriorating. He would come home from work too drained to engage with his wife and children, and weekends, which were once filled with family activities, had turned into time spent recovering from the week.

We began with a clear focus on outcomes. I asked J a simple but powerful question: What do you want? He realised that he'd been prioritising the wrong things and that he wanted more than just to feel physically better, he wanted to show up fully for his family, rediscover joy in his life and have a sense of purpose again.

With this new found clarity, we devised a practical, manageable plan. The first step was regular movement. J hadn't been prioritising exercise, so we introduced a balanced routine that included cardio and strength training. This helped him regain physical energy while also serving as a stress reliever.

At the same time we cleaned up his diet. J's nutrition had slipped due to his hectic lifestyle—too many processed foods, caffeine and irregular eating patterns. I replaced these with a sustainable plan focusing on whole foods, healthy fats, and lean proteins, which gave him sustained energy throughout the day and supported fat loss.

But beyond the physical, we worked deeply on his emotional and psychological wellbeing. J had been going through the motions, disconnected from his values and purpose. Together, we explored what really mattered to him—family, meaningful work, and personal growth. I also introduced him to various tools to help deepen his connection with his wife and children. We worked on active listening and being present with his family, and he started setting clear boundaries between work and home life, ensuring he had the time and energy to invest in the relationships that mattered most.

Physically, J's energy levels had skyrocketed. He dropped several inches from his waistline, which gave him an immediate confidence boost.

But the real breakthrough went far beyond the physical changes. J began making time for his family, showing up in the evenings and at weekends fully present, and engaging with his kids in ways he hadn't in years. The improved communication with his wife also led to a stronger, more intimate relationship.

This book is going to break it all down for you, step by step, providing you not only a clear understanding of what's going on for us at this stage of life, but also to give you simple actionable steps to work with it: To optimise your hormone health, speed up your metabolism, boost your positive "can do" mindset and get your libido firing. My aim is to leave you feeling confident, more than ready to face the world and embrace whatever challenges it throws at you.

So, do you want to drift through in a malaise, living an apathetic midlife? Or, do you want an energised, thriving, power packed life, regardless of what stage you are at?

I promise you there's nothing impossible for you to do. The steps are simple. They're achievable. The results are fantastic. You literally have nothing to lose and everything to gain.

We have already established that men aged 50 to 54 represent the highest suicide cohort. Men overall are less likely to maintain social relationships during midlife and even if they do, they're less likely to be vulnerable and open up about how they're feeling, instead suffering in silence.

Men are less likely than women to seek professional help, be that medical or therapy.

Men are more likely than women to turn to alcohol and/or drugs as a crutch and to indulge in risky behaviour.

Guys, we are literally killing ourselves and it has to stop!

At the same time we have life's pressures – juggling careers, relationships, finances, ageing parents, older children, what's going on in the world...

This stress has a huge impact on our physical, mental and psychological health as we'll see.

Finally, we need to address what's going on with testosterone as we age. Hardly anyone has heard of andropause. Have you? Chances are that you haven't, yet as a man, at some point from your 40s onwards you're going to feel at least some of the effects of it.

We've made huge leaps forward in recent years talking about menopause and making information and treatment more available for women, which is an excellent thing, but there is still so much to do in this area.

I'm fortunate to be at the cutting edge of menopause education. I go out to organisations and talk to male employees about menopause and how to be better allies in work, and to support their partners and women in their life. It's great that we're busting the taboos around the subject, having open conversations, and making strides forward.

One thing that always strikes me, though, is the almost complete lack of awareness about andropause and the impact of declining testosterone on men, as well as the knock on effect it can have on careers, relationships and wellbeing.

A recent UK survey found that 82% of men aged 40 to 55 had at least one symptom of andropause, but despite that, 78% were unaware of the existence of the term.

> *"A recent UK survey found that 82% of men aged 40 to 55 had at least one symptom of andropause, but despite that 78% were unaware of the existence of the term."*

Shockingly, despite the research available, andropause is still largely undiscussed, undiagnosed, or even dismissed simply as "age related testosterone decline". In fact, although low testosterone is a driver of andropause and its symptoms, there are many other factors at play.

We can't simply dismiss it as an age related phenomenon to be quietly dealt with personally.

Remember, until recently menopause wasn't widely discussed, women largely suffered in silence with little research given to understand the lifestyle factors that could help manage the effects. Instead, antidepressants became a popular prescription for treatment.

Whilst we still have a long way to go, we are turning the corner when it comes to menopause. Companies are introducing menopause policies, there are books, forums, support groups and of course HRT, along with a greater understanding of how to manage the effects.

We're at the same point now with andropause we were with menopause 20 years ago. No one really wants to talk about it and it's seen as just a by-product of ageing.

Many doctors don't recognise it, the NHS doesn't want to treat it. As a middle-aged man, if you go to your doctor presenting the symptoms you're far more likely to be dismissed by being told what you're experiencing is simply a sign of ageing than you are to have a conversation about what could be going on for you hormonally.

In fact, the most requested test for men from their GP is the 'Tired All The Time' test (TATT) which screens for a range of issues via a blood test. Incredibly, it doesn't screen for testosterone levels!

Like many menopausal women have experienced, you might be offered antidepressants – but you're not depressed! There's a hormonal basis for the way you feel, and for what's happening to you physically.

We're going to cover this in more detail in later chapters, but here's an overview: The male primary sex hormone is testosterone. This peaks in our 20s then declines at a steady rate of 1 to 3% per year, which doesn't sound a lot, but by the time you're in your 50s, you could have testosterone levels 30% to 50% lower than in your 20s.

The impact can be further amplified by things like poor diet, lack of exercise, poor sleep, stress and pollutants, the list goes on.

Andropause can be a confusing and difficult stage of life for men.

Symptoms such as decreased libido, erectile dysfunction, fatigue and depression can leave men feeling lost and uncertain. These are symptoms that tend to be dismissed as simply ageing, or down to stress or depression. Yes, these factors can play a role but it goes deeper.

There are treatments available, but more importantly there are many simple lifestyle strategies you can adopt to make a real positive difference to your life. That is exactly what this book is for.

I'm on a mission to bring awareness to the issues men face at midlife, including andropause, so that you can stop suffering in silence and stop mentally beating yourself up for things like lack of energy and low libido. You can get rid of that nagging feeling that your body is letting you down, and understand that there's actually a whole load of hormonal changes going on from around 40 years onwards that can affect you mentally, physically and emotionally.

I want us to open up the conversation between each other so we can talk about these things openly, without embarrassment or fear. Guys, this is your health, your happiness and your life. Let's start sharing and talking. You can even use this book as a conversation opener if you'd like.

# WHAT YOU CAN EXPECT FROM THIS BOOK

You now have in your hands a guide for men going through this stage of life. It provides a comprehensive overview of midlife issues and of andropause, including its causes, symptoms and available treatments.

It offers a simple 30-day kickstart programme designed to help you manage your symptoms and improve your overall wellbeing. This programme has been carefully crafted to include practical advice and strategies for managing symptoms, as well as information on available treatments and resources.

It's an actionable plan that gives you the tools you need to make positive changes in your lives and lay down long term foundations. The best part is, it's easy to follow.

How we face midlife as men, and how we get the most from it, embracing it with positivity, is something we need to be discussing and taking action on. When you consider the human and financial cost, this is something we DO need to be talking about.

Men in their 50s are now most likely to leave employment and the highest suicide cohort is midlife men. While that is not of course solely due to andropause, can we really say that the confusion, shift in identity, and feeling of betrayal from our own body and mind isn't playing a part in feelings of anxiety and depression, or contributing to relationship break ups and poor job performance?

In regards to the UK, there is research that shows 82% of men have at least one sign of andropause, even though more than two thirds (78%) have never heard the term 'andropause'. A further UK study revealed that 65% of men aged 40–55 said they are also experiencing low energy levels, 30% have problems with their sleeping, weight gain (30%) and muscle and joint pain (30%) along with hair loss (27%), decreased libido (25%), and erectile dysfunction (20%).

Clearly we need to be doing more to raise awareness both of the condition, and the lifestyle adjustments we can make to help optimise our midlife experience.

We are going to briefly cover testosterone replacement therapy, and while it can be a help to some men diagnosed with low testosterone, just like HRT, it's not a magic bullet in itself. You'll still need to make the other lifestyle changes that we're going to cover in this book.

I guess if you're reading this book, chances are that you're a guy who's 40 plus and has started to wonder if there might not be an underlying reason for the way you're feeling, and more importantly if there's something you can do about it. I'm here to give you the answers to both those questions. Before we get any further I want to give you the good news – there is plenty you can do about it without making massive changes to your lifestyle.

Perhaps areas of your life like your relationship are suffering, but you're not really sure why.

## CASE STUDY: **STEPHEN (46)**

Stephen's relationship with his wife was strained due to frequent arguments, communication breakdowns, and decreased intimacy, made worse by his work stress, inducing irritability and mood swings.

We worked on communication skills and tools, on stress reduction techniques and practice, on looking at things outside of work that Stephen could focus on to reduce work tension and over time their relationship improved significantly. They regained intimacy and harmony in their marriage and Stephen felt way less stressed, and able to face life full on again with a spring in his step. Getting a handle on stress (which can be so toxic) is vital, and we're going to cover that too as it also impacts our hormone health.

If that sounds familiar then you are in the right place. In this book I'm going to share some really great information that you can action straightaway. Stuff that can make a difference to you in a matter of weeks, and no, this doesn't involve harsh workouts or restrictive, weird diets. This is all practical advice that's easy to put into place.

We'll cover myths and mistakes, which is where so many people go wrong and waste time, money and energy. Then before we dive into hormones we're going to look at a crucial element that's so often overlooked, and that's the importance of aligning the mind and body.

We're going to take a look at midlife male hormones, the huge impact of stress and then we're going to get into the action steps. Specifically we're going to cover the importance of movement, of nutrition, of building a success mindset and creating emotional resilience. Finally, we'll cover the importance of accountability.

In the second part of the book I'm going to lay out a simple three part 30-day programme for you:

- Workouts
- Nutrition
- Mindset

Read the first part first so you understand the theory, then dive into the programme and start taking action.

What I'd love for you by the end of this book is that you not only have a clear idea of what's going with your hormones, an understanding of the many ways that's affecting you, but you understand what to do to perform at your full potential. I want you excited by the possibilities, motivated to go on that journey: Because it is possible, and it's possible for you.

To perform at your full potential, you might need to adjust your diet, you might need to change your exercise (or even just get started) and you will certainly need to focus your mindset, but I will guide you every step of the way.

So join me on this journey of discovery as we empower men to take control of their health and improve their quality of life during andropause. This is not just another book on andropause, it's a comprehensive guide that provides a clear path for readers to follow and gives them the tools they need to make positive changes in their lives.

# About Me

*I'm James. I'm one half of something called the Midlife Mentors, a midlife health and performance brand my wife and I originally started as a podcast at the end of 2019. Alongside the original podcast, it has since evolved into a health coaching brand that's helped thousands of people transform their lives. We work alongside blue chip corporates and operate transformational retreats in the UK and Spain.*

Prior to this, I founded the luxury transformational retreat company 38 Degrees North in 2012, again working with thousands of clients on physical health, mindset and nutrition. More about all that in a moment, because how I started out on this path and what happened is important.

Back at school when I was very young I was that overweight kid that was picked last for sports – and tried to avoid them. It didn't help that I was sent to a boarding school where there was a big emphasis on sports, and living at the school itself, there was no respite by going home. Free time was filled with sports too. In a strange twist of fate, being sent to that school that prioritised sport was my turnaround. I had to learn to love it, the weight came off, I became athletic and I discovered the gym as a way to feel more confident.

However those early years left me with body dysmorphia issues. Even at university I can remember eating small salads, scared about getting fat, when I should have been gobbling down big meals. I still lacked confidence and that didn't really come to me until I pushed myself further outside my comfort zone by travelling around the USA on my own in my early twenties. Thankfully by learning more, by applying the training and nutrition tools that I had, by putting myself in situations where I had to rely on myself, I eventually came through this phase.

At university I studied Social Psychology and I went on to complete a Masters in Applied Psychology and a MBA. I'm a qualified personal trainer with additional qualifications in coaching, NLP, sports nutrition, gut health, hypnosis and hormone health. I also have a diploma in Jungian Psychology and I'm a menopause practitioner: I go into organisations to talk to them about the impact of menopause and andropause and help them define strategies around them. I love learning! Fun fact: I'm also a qualified stand up paddle instructor.

So that's me, that's the life experience and the tool kit I bring to the table. When I stepped away from the corporate world to launch 38 Degrees North I wanted to combine all of these elements: psychology and mindset, nutrition, training and coaching, with the focus on midlife, gut health and hormones.

I'm a massive believer in the importance of mastering the mind (too many people focus on the "external", the nutrition and training, without addressing limiting beliefs, behaviours and self identity). This is why I believe Claire and I have such success with our clients, because we bed in habits that support lasting change, as well as immediate results.

As I've said already, it's crucial to align your body and mind and yet this is what I see people not doing, over and over again.

They feel like they're putting on weight, they don't like what they see in the mirror, so they opt for the diet, they go for the workout, but they're not adjusting their internal state, they are not working on their mindset.

I can't emphasise enough that these elements have got to work together. What I see over and over again, is people get the body going but they neglect the mindset and then it doesn't work. It's not going to get you to your full potential if you don't engage both body and mind.

As you're reading this in 2025, I'll be heading towards my 53rd birthday. I still have the same 32 inch waist I had in my early twenties, I'm lean (I stay between 12–14% body fat), I'm energised, I have a great libido. I'm positive about life.

I don't obsess about what I eat, I don't spend hours in the gym, I get out and enjoy life, drinks, burgers, parties... it's just that I know how to work in line with my mind and body to maintain my results, and boy, does that make life so much more satisfying.

One last thing about me, and this is not a "poor me" tale, but it's so you know it hasn't all been an easy cake walk. In 2014 my wife and partner of over 15 years left me suddenly. My confidence was rock bottom once again. I felt worthless. I was trying to make sense of what had happened, run a business serving others and struggling to identify who I now was. We lost our beautiful home in London as neither of us could afford to buy the other out. Suddenly

I'd lost my wife and my home, I felt on the scrap heap of life and destined to be alone.

That triggered lots of old destructive patterns and behaviours. I entered a spiral of unhealthy relationships with myself and with others, I punished myself by overtraining my body and drinking too much to blot out the pain.

My self confidence was shot.

Why I'm sharing this is because I came back from that, and I was already in my 40s when that happened. Literally, I was 42 and I thought I was all washed up. I thought no one would want me. I didn't even want myself. I didn't like my body. I couldn't form relationships. I was in pain and in a destructive spiral.

Gradually I figured it out and applied what I knew, using my tools on myself.

Here's where I am now:

Running a multi award retreat and coaching business serving thousands of clients. I'm an author. I'm a speaker. I'm regularly asked to commentate in the press. I have a wonderful marriage now, a thriving business and I believe in myself. I get to talk to women about menopause and to men about andropause in corporate environments.

Our podcast The Midlife Mentors (do check it out) is in the top 1.5% of global podcasts and I'm lucky enough to split my time between London and Spain.

Most importantly, I'm a midlifer just like you. I've been in a corporate rat race. I'm your age. I know how it is. I know the ups. I've experienced the crashing downs. I know the demands on you, the pressures, time, money, family, career.

If I can do it, then you can do it, and I'm going to give you the tools to do it.

Are you ready?

# Things You Probably Didn't Know But Should

*Here's a big shock for you... Andropause doesn't exist!*

What? What am I reading then?

Well, let me explain, as more people have started talking about andropause there's also been a growth in the anti-andropause movement. If you search online for 'andropause' you're bound to find comments from 'experts', sometimes medical doctors, saying that we shouldn't use the term andropause as it equates too closely with menopause and muddies the waters...

Sadly you will also find some menopause proponents who say the same thing. There are a few reasons why this happens. Firstly, yes there is concern that a focus on andropause might detract from menopause. But they are not mutually exclusive, talking about one doesn't take anything away from the other. In fact, because menopause and andropause are occurring at similar life stages and most couples are in similar age relationships, we should be talking about both.

Secondly there seems to be a drive to downplay andropause as having less impact on less men than menopause does on women. Again, this is true, but if we conservatively estimate that low testosterone is impacting in the region of 20% of men aged 40 to 65, then that would be approximately 1.4 million men in the UK alone, and some 4 million in the USA. That's a lot of men suffering with symptoms and having careers, health and relationships impacted.

These experts will say that low testosterone is very different to menopause in women. Yes it is. But it still exists.

They'll also point out that all women go through menopause at some point and so will be likely to show the symptoms and be affected. Also true, but this comes back to the arguments of having two gender specific processes and not trying to detract from menopause by using the term andropause.

The truth is that menopause is hard for the majority of women, because the drop in oestrogen (their primary sex hormone) happens a) in a relatively short window of time compared to male's drop in testosterone, so symptoms are likely to be more pronounced. And b) because that drop is also accompanied by wild fluctuations in hormone levels, again leading to more pronounced symptoms.

However, some women do go through menopause with hardly any symptoms. The difference is they are in the minority, whereas for andropause, men who are experiencing symptoms are in the minority. That still doesn't mean we should dismiss it though.

For men, because the decline in testosterone levels are gradual, the symptoms are more gradual so can be harder to spot, but once you do start feeling them, then you will notice them.

At the end of the day it's purely an argument in semantics. If you want to call it andropause, you should, if you want to call it age related testosterone decline, low testosterone, hypogonadism (actually a term for very low testosterone levels at any age), then feel free, but let's start recognising that yes, while it is different and distinct from menopause, like menopause, it is driven by a decline in our primary sex hormones, and that it is likely to occur at midlife into late midlife.

Also, just like menopause, it's not just about testosterone; other hormones and neurotransmitter levels are also changing, stress also plays a huge role, but more on that shortly.

# The State We're In... All About Testosterone

*Our testosterone is in crisis. Yep, testosterone levels have been falling since the 1980s, with average levels declining by about 1% per year. This means, for example, that a 60-year-old man in 2004 had testosterone levels 17% lower than those of a 60-year-old in 1987.*

This also means that a greater proportion of men in 2024 would have had below-normal testosterone levels than in 1987.

A 22-year-old today has less testosterone than a 70-year-old 50 years ago.

*"A 22-year-old today has less testosterone than a 70-year-old 50 years ago."*

Sperm production has fallen 59% since the 1970s and sperm counts fell on average by 1.2% per year between 1973 to 2018, but since 2000 have accelerated to 2.6% per year.

It is estimated that in 1995 there were over 152 million men worldwide who experienced ED; the projections for 2025 show a prevalence of approximately 322 million with ED, an increase of nearly 170 million men.

In a 2016 study, the average 20- to 34-year-old man could apply 98 pounds of force with a right-handed grip, down from 117 pounds by a man of the same age in 1985.

So we're also getting physically weaker. Then of course there's the shifting role of men in society. Go back 50 years or so and society and culture were very different. A man's role was more defined, masculine traits were accepted, men tended to be the main breadwinners and to focus on their careers as a way of providing for their families.

Today the role and expected behaviour of men in society is less clear. The workplace has shifted from traditional labour based roles like factory work and manufacturing that favoured men, to more service based that tend to be more dominated by women. Young men have fallen behind women in education levels and tend to drop out of the work environment more, perhaps echoing that sense of, if not a lack of, certainly a confusion of role or purpose.

Has testosterone declined in response to a changing world, or has the world shaped around men with lower testosterone? Or is it both?

One thing is certain, testosterone levels have fallen, but why?

It's complex.

Factors include higher rates of obesity (raised body fat lowers testosterone production), less exercise, more environmental toxins, such as pesticides, parabens and chemicals common in household products like phthalates and bisphenol A, along with more oestrogen in our water.

We do less physical work and even the types of relationships we have could impact testosterone levels (stable relationships tend to lower testosterone). So, there are a lot of factors at play. What matters is that we acknowledge it and do something about it.

# WHAT DOESN'T HELP IS A LACK OF MEDICAL AWARENESS

Doctors will typically get anything between two to four hours training on menopause during their entire years of training. They don't get any on andropause. Of course they are aware of testosterone and the symptoms of low testosterone, but this is often viewed as a specific condition (hypogonadism) rather than looking at the broader view of what could be happening for mens' testosterone levels as they age.

Which means if you go to see your GP, unless you're very fortunate, they aren't likely to diagnose your symptoms as being due to low testosterone.

So top tip, if you are going to see your doctor about how you're feeling, do bring up low testosterone and ask if you can have a blood test to check your testosterone levels.

It is worth noting here that whilst blood tests can be useful, they are only showing you what's going on at a particular moment in time, so ideally you'd want a series in order to get an idea of how your testosterone levels are fluctuating. Unfortunately this is often not possible, so you may be stuck with the one test.

These thresholds from the British Society for Sexual Medicine (BSSM) [8] might be useful to help you understand your results:

Testosterone levels greater than 15 nmol/L typically don't require treatment

Testosterone levels between 8 – 12 nmol/L (or 8–14 nmol/L if you have pre-diabetes) might require a trial of testosterone replacement therapy (TRT) if there are symptoms of testosterone deficiency. In these cases, it's useful to check free testosterone levels, often with other male sex hormones.

Testosterone levels less than 8 nmol/L usually require treatment.

Just to confuse things further... you'll get a reading back of total testosterone and free testosterone. About 98% of our testosterone is bound, meaning it's already being utilised, the 2% to 5% free is what's available to us, so it could be possible to have normal total testosterone levels but low free testosterone, in which case you could have the symptoms of low testosterone.

Normal levels of free testosterone are anything above 0.300nmol/l and an optimal range is above 0.45nmol/l.

In summary, if your total testosterone is low, or if your total testosterone is okay but your free testosterone is low, then it's time to start the lifestyle adjustments laid out in this book, and you may also want to consider medical treatment.

However, remember, medical treatments often need to be supported by positive changes in your lifestyle too, in order to reap the full benefits. If you opt for testosterone replacement therapy (TRT) but your lifestyle remains suboptimal for your testosterone to thrive, the benefits are not going to be as great as they could be by addressing those lifestyle factors.

## Testosterone Myths And Stigma

Over the years testosterone has earned something of a bad reputation, primarily due to its association with enhancing performance in sport, and in particular with body builders using it to put on muscle. We hear phrases like "roid rage" and if someone's aggravated we might comment that "their testosterone's a bit high".

So let's dispel some of the stigma, but first acknowledge that yes, if you take testosterone at high levels, it will improve your sporting performance and help you put on muscle, but the side effects include acne, mood swings, excessive body hair growth, head hair loss, heart muscle damage, prostate enlargement, low sperm count, low libido, testicular shrinkage and erectile dysfunction. When we introduce testosterone into the body externally, it will compensate by aromatising testosterone into oestrogen, which is why formation of breast tissue can be another side effect.

However, if you're naturally raising your testosterone through lifestyle adjustments, or on a medically prescribed therapy you're not going to suffer from these symptoms.

Put simply the myths and stigma come from abuse of testosterone, yet interestingly it's this stigma that has persisted. It's time for that to end. At midlife we want to ensure that our testosterone is within a healthy range so that both our health and quality of life are optimised.

## Testosterone Benefits

Having optimised testosterone levels will mean that you have more energy, you'll find it easier to build or maintain muscle, burn fat and have a healthy libido. There's also a positive impact on mental health in terms of focus and confidence.

## Treatments

This book is not about treatments and not about TRT. It's about making simple adjustments to your lifestyle that pay big benefits and will help you with andropause. However, you may already be in a position where your testosterone levels are low enough that you want to consider TRT as an option.

If you decide to go down this road, please do your research. TRT is transformative for many men, but it's not for everyone and there are side effects you need to be aware of.

The main one being that if you go onto TRT you will shut down your own testosterone production, so this is a lifetime decision. It will also affect your fertility. There can also be contraindications around prostate issues, certain cancers and cardiovascular conditions, so do your research.

If you're going to opt for TRT then you'll also have a variety of options for taking the testosterone, including implants, injections and creams. All have pros and cons.

Finally remember, it's not a magic bullet – you still need to do everything outlined in this book to optimise your health. I'd rather you give the lifestyle adjustments a good go for three months to see the improvement, before deciding on TRT.

## But... It's Not Just About Testosterone

This phase of life is not just about testosterone. As we hit midlife a number of hormones and neurotransmitters change. I call this the portfolio effect. These changes impact us physically and psychologically, so it's important to understand them and know what we can do to work with them.

First up we're becoming more insulin resistant, which essentially means we're less efficient at processing the food and drinks we consume for energy. In turn this means that we're more likely to store excess energy as fat.

It's also worth noting that as we age our digestive system becomes less efficient at extracting nutrients from our food. If twenty year old you and fifty year old you sat down and ate exactly the same steak, twenty year old you is going to get a lot more protein and nutrients from that steak than fifty year old you, so what and how we eat is important.

Let's look at an example; if an average 500g rump steak has around 160g of protein, we can generally absorb around 50% of that protein. Obviously there a number of factors that affect that (genetics, gut health, other food in the meal, hydration etc..), but a younger you could potentially utilise 51% or around 82g of that protein, an older version of you might only be able to utilise around 45% or 72g of that protein. That might not sound like a big difference, but over every meal, day after day, the difference sure adds up.

Linked to our ability to utilise nutrients effectively is our gut health. Our gut is home to billions of living organisms called biomes. These organisms play a role in metabolism and, via the production of neurotransmitters, our mood and cognition. Our gut is linked to our brain via the Vagus nerve which allows for some of the fastest signalling in our body – we call this the gut/brain connection. So we want to ensure we're optimising our gut health for both metabolism and mood.

The levels of the leptin, our satiety hormone, decline with age, so we're more likely to overeat. Processed and ultra processed foods seem to fail to trigger leptin so if our diet is high in these we're more likely to overeat. They are also inflammatory to the gut, body and brain.

Levels of Human Growth Hormone peak in our adolescence and then decline. HGH helps us build new tissue and maintain what we have, so together with declining testosterone, this is why we start to lose muscle mass as we age. We need to be doing regular resistance workouts to counteract this.

We have cells called mitochondria in the body that provide us with energy. These too decline with age, meaning we have less energy, however regular exercise can help boost and maintain elevated levels.

Finally research into our feel good neurotransmitter serotonin suggests it declines as we age. This means we can be more prone to low mood or anxiety. There's also evidence linking low levels to cognitive disorders like dementia and Alzheimer's. Again, the right diet and exercise can help keep serotonin levels boosted.

This isn't an exhaustive list, but it does give you an idea of some of the main changes Going on at midlife and beyond – no wonder it can feel so challenging at times!

Throw low testosterone into the mix and what do you have? Potentially weight gain, low energy, low libido, low drive, anxiety, loss of confidence, apathy...

The good news is, it doesn't have to be this way!

## A Short Word On Getting Your Prostate Checked

As men, something we need to be aware of is our risk of prostate cancer. Incidences of this type of cancer have increased 53% since the 1990s in the UK and it's the most common cancer in males in the UK, accounting for 28% of all new cancer cases in males. It mainly affects men over 50, with the risk increasing with age. In the UK, about 1 in 8 men will get prostate cancer in their lifetime.

The prostate is a small gland about the size of a walnut that sits under the bladder and around the urethra, and its role is to help with the production of semen. A sign that you may have an issue which could be an enlarged prostate (which is common as men age) or a sign of prostate cancer include needing to pee more frequently, frequent urgent needs to urinate, hesitancy when urinating, straining, weak flow or feeling your bladder isn't emptying fully.

If you're over 50 even if you don't have these symptoms it's a good idea to get your prostate checked, and yes it did used to involve a rather intrusive probe from your doctor or a nurse but these days you can also get a simple blood test (PSA) that will screen for signs of prostate issues. Do get yourself checked out, it might save your life.

# STRESS IS KILLING YOUR LIBIDO AND MAKING YOU FAT!

### CASE STUDY: **BILL (44)**

Bill was a 44-year-old high-powered lawyer, already juggling the demands of a busy career while being a time-poor father of three. He was up for a major promotion at work, a role that would require even more energy, focus and stamina. However, Bill wasn't feeling at his best. He had gained a little weight over the past few years, his clothes no longer fit as they used to and his self-confidence had taken a hit. With a stressful job and frequent client meals, Bill knew he didn't have time for a fad diet or an extreme fitness regime. He needed a tailored, realistic approach that took into account the unique challenges of midlife men.

Understanding Bill's packed schedule and high-stakes career, we focused on a plan that was sustainable, practical, and effective. We started with a nutritional plan designed specifically for him, one that allowed him to navigate client dinners and busy workdays without derailing his progress. Rather than restrictive dieting, we focused on making smart choices at meals, improving the quality of his food and finding ways to keep his energy levels stable throughout the day.

In addition, we implemented short, focused training sessions that Bill could easily fit into his schedule. These sessions targeted fat loss, muscle maintenance and overall fitness without requiring hours in the gym. These efficient workouts gave Bill the physical benefits he needed while fitting seamlessly into his lifestyle.

Beyond the physical, we placed a strong emphasis on mindset. Bill's work was mentally demanding and his responsibilities at home were equally intense. We incorporated daily practices to help him develop a resilient, focused mindset, including stress management techniques and mindfulness strategies. This helped Bill not only stay disciplined with his health goals but also manage the pressures of his work and personal life more effectively.

In just a few weeks, Bill saw a dramatic transformation. He successfully lost the weight he wanted to lose and as a result, his clothes fit him better, boosting his confidence. The physical changes were obvious, but more importantly, Bill felt better about himself. His energy levels improved and he developed a sharper focus at work.

> With his newfound energy and confidence, Bill approached the promotion process with a sense of empowerment. He felt not only capable of handling the added responsibilities of the role but excited about taking it on. Bill's hard work paid off, he landed the promotion he'd been working towards.
>
> Perhaps most telling was Bill's own reflection on the programme.
>
> *"The difference with your programme is that you understand what people are going through psychologically, emotionally, spiritually and physically. You've nailed it!"*

Before we move on, there's one final hormone I want to talk about. The stress hormone cortisol. When we're stressed we fire a cocktail of hormones, one of those is cortisol. Now cortisol's role is as a get up and go signaller. It's designed to spike in the morning then decline through the day.

However in today's high stress environment what can happen is that it spikes in the morning, then carries on rising through the day as we encounter stressful situations. Our stress response is designed for physical confrontations, but our brain doesn't distinguish between real physical threats, or perceived threats, like an angry email, bad news and so on.

So we get a physiological response geared for physical action: heart rate and blood pressure increase to oxygenate the blood, non-essential (from the standpoint of the immediate stress event) bodily systems shut down: digestion, immune system, reproductive system.

We get a narrow focus on the perceived threat often leading to us missing what else is going on around us. We have decreased sensitivity to pain, our serotonin levels drop…

Those are the immediate effects. Over time consistently raised cortisol actually makes us hold onto more body fat, particularly in the abdominal area, makes us more anxious, can start to break down muscle tissue, impact our libido, impact our confidence and crucially decrease levels of testosterone.

That's because both testosterone and cortisol are made from the same "mother" hormone pregnenolone, so if you're making more cortisol, there's less pregnenolone available for testosterone.

So, cortisol on its own is bad enough, but at a time of life where you could be struggling with low testosterone, stress is going to lower it still further.

This means that getting a handle on stress is crucial and we'll be covering what you can do to help manage your stress more effectively.

# Understanding Andropause And Its Impacts

*By now you probably have a good idea of what andropause is, but let's briefly cover off exactly what it is, and the impacts it can have.*

Andropause is a natural phase in a man's life characterised by a decline in testosterone levels. It differs from other male health issues in that it's a gradual hormonal shift rather than a sudden cessation of hormone production. Unlike menopause in women, which involves a clear cessation of menstruation, andropause occurs more subtly in men, typically starting in their late 40s to early 50s. While testosterone decline is a significant factor, andropause involves a range of physical, emotional, and psychological changes beyond hormonal shifts.

During andropause, testosterone levels gradually decrease, impacting various bodily functions. This decline in testosterone production can lead to physical changes such as reduced muscle mass, increased body fat, decreased bone density, and changes in hair growth patterns.

Additionally, hormonal fluctuations can contribute to symptoms like fatigue, decreased libido, erectile dysfunction, and sleep disturbances. The hormonal shifts also play a role in mood changes, cognition, and overall wellbeing.

Andropause can manifest through a variety of symptoms, including persistent fatigue, diminished energy levels, mood swings, irritability, decreased motivation, and a decline in libido or sexual desire. Men might also experience difficulties in achieving or maintaining erections, which can affect sexual function and intimacy. Other symptoms may include memory problems, sleep disturbances, and decreased physical endurance.

Diagnosing andropause involves a comprehensive assessment of symptoms and medical history. Healthcare providers may perform blood tests to measure testosterone levels and other hormone levels.

Additionally, a physical examination and discussion of symptoms are crucial for accurate diagnosis. Differential diagnosis helps rule out other medical conditions with similar symptoms. A healthcare professional's evaluation and interpretation of symptoms, hormone levels, and physical examination findings contribute to a proper diagnosis of andropause.

## Impacts

As you can imagine, with such wide ranging symptoms that affect your body, mind, emotions and libido the impacts of andropause can be both significant and multi-layered.

## Physical

Andropause affects men both physically and emotionally. The physical changes encompass alterations in body composition, energy levels, sexual function, and overall vitality. These changes can significantly impact a man's quality of life and wellbeing.

Typically men will lose muscle mass, and put on more body fat, particularly around their midsection. This in turn can have a psychological and emotional impact with lowered body confidence, reduced willingness to be intimate and psychosexual issues along with loss of libido.

## Emotional And Psychological Impact

The emotional and psychological effects of andropause can include mood swings, anxiety, depression, irritability, and decreased self-esteem. This is why it's vital to not just focus on the physical side of things, but invest in your mental health as well by having coping strategies and mental health support to help navigate these emotional challenges.

## Relationships And Communication

Andropause can also affect relationships and communication dynamics. Changes in mood, libido, and physical energy levels may impact intimacy and communication with partners, family, and friends. If you're in a relationship with someone going through menopause, then the impact can be huge.

You can see that there's a lot going on here, there's a lot to unpack. Thankfully the solutions are simple to implement. If you're willing. If you start to think that it might be too hard, remind yourself of the alternative and ask which reality you want to live: apathy or purpose?

# Who Is This Book For?

*It's for you. It's for you if you feel like you're struggling. That you're under pressure at work and at home. That there are things happening with your body you don't like and you're not sure how to fix them.*

Maybe you're feeling under constant time pressure, perhaps you've got an unhealthy relationship with food or drink, maybe both. It could be that you've stopped believing in yourself, that you've got to that point where you're sleepwalking through life apathetic about the future.

It's for you if you don't like what you see in the mirror, or if you swing between all or nothing, in work, in fitness, in anything... this is so common, you know.

How many times have you said to yourself, "This is it. I'm going to do it, this is the week I'm going to change it." Then comes the, "I just can't be bothered."

This is for you if you seem to self sabotage and never stay consistent. It's for you if your relationships are suffering. Those could be your work relationships, your work performance or it could be your relationships at home with your partner and your family, maybe both of those...

It's for you if, most importantly, you want to do something to change all this.

Let me tell you this, changing all the above isn't as hard as you think, AND it's a damn sight easier than doing nothing, because here's the thing, if you're not taking steps to change things, then you're not standing still, you're going backwards.

Knowing you can implement simple change is a powerful confidence booster in itself. There's also this... if you do nothing what do the next 3 months, 6 months, a year, two years look like?

> ## CASE STUDY: **DAVID (52)**
>
> David was experiencing frequent mood swings, irritability, and difficulty concentrating, affecting his performance at work and relationships with colleagues. He had a potential promotion coming up and felt that not only did he not have the energy and focus, but that he wasn't in a good place from a work relationships perspective. We worked on his mindset with simple tools, coached him on communication styles, and tweaked his nutrition and exercise. Over time, David noticed a significant reduction in mood swings and irritability. He became more focused at work and found it easier to maintain positive relationships with colleagues and got his promotion. Life will always throw us curve balls but knowing how to deal with them is what gives us power.

So let's talk about what's needed from you...

My clients have something in common. They're action takers. Now that might sound odd given that my clients are all successful men, but how many men do you know (maybe yourself included) that are action takers in business, their careers, finance, relationships, but neglect to take action on their health? I can tell you, plenty...

So the people I work with are smart, they take responsibility. They do the hard yards mentally and physically, they're consistent and they're in it for the long haul, because yes you can get results fast (and you will) but it is about the long haul and sustainable results.

In this book I can and will give you so many tips and tricks that you can put into action, but the keyword there is action. I can't wave a magic wand and do it for you.

Just like reading a Haynes manual doesn't make you a mechanic, reading this won't get you in shape mentally and physically unless you implement it. But you're going to, because why would you not when it's easy and the results massively outweigh the effort?

Listen, if you follow what I tell you, you are going to get results.

Those results will come relatively quickly, but this is not for people looking for fast solutions or fad fixes. I'm not about the diet or the miracle workout or the supplement.

Here's the problem with today's society – unrealistic expectations. If you're not prepared to put the work in, then you can't expect to see the results. People are not willing to keep an open mind. People aren't prepared for the mental reps as well as physical reps. I get this all the time. People say to me, "just give me a workout programme".

"No" is always my answer. We are interconnected beings and we need a holistic solution. We need to do the mindset work. Success is 80% psychology 20% mechanics.

The belief and behaviour work is so important and that's why I leverage my experience of a Master's in Psychology, Master Coach, NLP, this is the stuff that is going to change your life for the long term.

Since the 1950s, advertising has sold us a dream of everything being easier, simpler, faster. Sadly it's not always like that, especially when it comes to our health. Our culture reinforces often unrealistic body images for both men and women through mainstream media and social media, and in fact social media drives us to compare our lives to others – even though they themselves are often presenting a false narrative, a curated version of themselves.

That's why we need to be realistic in our expectations, and take responsibility for our outcomes. When we do it's amazing what we can achieve.

If you're ready to take responsibility for yourself and you're willing to be consistent and committed, then the answer is here in your hands. Let's do this.

# Let's Talk About Those Big Midlife Challenges...

*There's that word "midlife". Is it a dirty word? How does it make you feel? One person told me that no man wants to think that they are middle aged, but on the flip side I've met a load of men who tell me this is the best part of their life so far.*

Midlife is just a label. Think of it as shorthand for the time in your life somewhere between 40 and 60 or so. It can be such a rewarding time, we have so many positives. By now you have a career, a reputation, character...

You know yourself, you have confidence in your abilities. You're probably financially secure, maybe have a family, but here's the thing, I bet you care less what other people think about you now, and that's a good thing because it means you're open.

Our 40s and beyond can be a second act we embrace with joy, and they should be (and I'm going to show you how) BUT... and there is a but, we do face some age related challenges.

So what are the challenges we face at this time in life?

First up, understand that a lot of these aren't directly your fault. There's chemical processes going on in the body that cause these things.

We've already covered these, but then add in juggling your career, ageing parents, growing kids, finances, your relationship, the state of the world...

No wonder we can feel overwhelmed. But you know, that's okay, let's find our way out of that overwhelm so we can live a better life. One thing I always say is that knowing where we are gives us a starting point.

So if you're feeling under pressure, stressed, overwhelmed, that's fine, it's also normal. Here's where I see people going wrong. Men try to fix this by either:

a) Ignoring it completely and doing nothing (newsflash – that ain't gonna work), or

b) Going into "man" mode and misdirecting their efforts with such things like focussing on work or a rigorous new workout routine, because they don't want to deal with the uncomfortable "internal stuff" like emotions and how they're feeling.

I get it, the declining physicality is scaring you, but beasting yourself may get you short term results (it won't get you long term ones) and is going to fix that other "icky" stuff you don't want to look at but that you know you really need to. Don't be afraid of your vulnerability. Embrace it.

Don't go down the workout route – you're just punishing yourself.

It just will not work. Hormonally, physiologically, you are a very different being to the one you were earlier in your life and you need a different approach, which I'm going to give you in this book.

First, let's look at a real life client, make sure we're setting ourselves realistic outcomes and look at some of the most common mistakes you could be making.

## CASE STUDY: **PAUL (42)**

So I'd love to briefly tell you about Paul, one of my clients, because what he was experiencing, and how we worked together will resonate with what you might be feeling, and show you that there's a way forward

When Paul came to me, he was outwardly successful, all of his ducks in a row. He's running his own business, very successful, obviously with his challenges through the pandemic like most of us, but coping and doing well. Paul's married, has two young kids, all should be rosy, but...

Despite all those outward trappings of success, that confidence in business, on a personal level he felt like he was on a downward spiral. He didn't feel like he was really firing on all cylinders, he was low on energy, and was lacking motivation at work.

He didn't feel like he was really connecting to his wife and to his kids when he was at home.

In fact at home he felt disengaged from his life, and this led to him drinking more than he wanted to, which in turn made most of the above worse and made him feel bad about himself.

I took Paul through an exercise I use with clients and he recognised that the thing he valued most was his relationship with his wife and kids, but that was where he was actually putting the least amount of energy and focus in his life. So there was a mismatch in the desired outcome and the inputs.

"Awareness precedes change" is a favourite mantra of mine, and this is one skill we can cultivate, to be honest with ourselves about where we are, what part we've played in getting there, where we want to be, and what we need to change.

It's about taking responsibility, and that also involves being vulnerable as often we'll need to admit where we got things wrong, where we're not showing up as the man we want to be, what our shortcomings are. We'll at least have to admit that to ourselves, but maybe to significant others in our lives too. That takes real courage, but the change you can drive from it is massive, that's why vulnerability is a super power.

You know what else? When combined with a dedication to change, it's also as sexy as hell to other people. If you hold your hands up and say "I recognise that I'm not showing up as I should do for myself or for you, and I'm sorry for that, but I'm committed to changing that," and you follow through, well...

> Paul did that, we worked on how he was going to communicate to his wife how he was going to step up, and as he followed through on his promise with his actions and deepened that communication with his wife, his relationship took on another dimension. She could see the man he was becoming and the fact he was sharing that with her built a whole new level of intimacy. In turn, this confidence improved Paul's relationship with his kids, with colleagues at work and his overall performance and happiness levels.

The key thing for Paul was, he recognised that something wasn't right and he wanted to make change.

Of course when he came to me as a possible solution he was apprehensive. He had a load of questions, as most clients do. Ultimately, all those questions come down to three things that everyone wants to know and they are:

- Is it going to work?
- What are we going to do?
- How much will it cost me in time and money?

The questions you have are likely the same for the information you're reading right now.

Well, is it going to work? Yes, if you follow what's laid out here, because like I say, I've got decades of experience, I've trained 1000s of clients, this categorically works. It's also a very research driven, evidence based approach. I'm always reading research papers, updating what we're doing to get clients and myself the results that we deserve. So yes, it works.

What we're going to do is laid out in the next few chapters of this book you're holding right now. We are going to give you some movement and break that down into the best way to train in the shortest time for long term results at 45 plus. We're talking lower body fat, increased muscle, more energy, better body shape and movement.

We're going give you some nutrition principles, so you don't have to overly restrict, can enjoy the foods you love and have a tool kit for long term healthy eating, reset your metabolism and increase your metabolic flexibility so that you're more efficient at burning food for energy.

We can basically shift between using either carbohydrates or fats as our energy source, and our ability to make this shift is our metabolic flexibility.

We should be burning carbohydrate energy through the day, and when we wake up in the morning, having fasted overnight we should be in a fat burning state (which is why fasted HIIT can be effective for fat loss with the right conditions). Of course if we're eating a lot of carbohydrates late in the day, then we're going to wake up still utilising carbohydrate energy, which is not what we want.

We're going to cover this in the programme section in more detail, but our aim should be to increase our metabolic flexibility and aim to awaken in that fat burning state.

We're also going to really dial in on the mindset of getting you thinking about your self identity, your goals, and your limiting beliefs that are holding you back. We're going to look at how we shift those beliefs to create a success based, positive mindset, and install new software that makes all of the above easier as you're working with yourself instead of against yourself.

# Reality And Outcomes

*Let's talk about reality and outcomes, because that gives us our starting point, and helps us set a realistic goal. The reality is that you would probably love a six pack, the reality is that you can have one, BUT, and it's a big but, you're probably going to be very unhappy getting to that point and then maintaining it.*

This is about setting realistic expectations. Here's an obvious one, the more body fat you're carrying right now, the longer it's going to take you to get down to somewhere approaching looking lean, because you have more fat to lose and there's only a certain rate you can lose it at.

Conversely though, your initial fat loss results are likely to be very fast, again, as you have more to lose. If you're currently already fairly lean, then shifting that last bit of body fat is probably going to be harder for you than someone very overweight making a dent in their body fat – because as we get down to lower body fat numbers it becomes harder to lose it.

That's why it's good to understand how much body fat you want to lose – what's your eventual body fat target? To help you with this I'm going to explain a concept I call the happiness window.

For most men, as a general rule of thumb, the abdominal muscles will start to show through the skin at somewhere around the 11 to 12% range of body fat. Of course this will vary depending on where you store fat on your body (and that's largely down to genetics but also partly hormones, so we will work on this). For example, I have friends whose body fat is pretty evenly distributed over their entire body, so they can have visible abs (just) as high as 14 to 15% body fat.

I store most of my fat on my stomach, with hardly any on the rest of my body, so even at 9% body fat I don't have super clearly defined abs – it's just the way I'm built.

I also know that above around 15–16% body fat I don't like my body, because I end up with a big stomach. I also know that getting to 10% or lower and keeping my body fat percentage there is miserable (and I look ill because my face goes gaunt). So my personal happiness window is between 11.5 and 13.5%.

I know that I like what I see, that I can maintain that really easily with exercise and managing carbs, but still enjoying burgers, pizzas, beers and the like within reason. So I feel good, I like how I look, and I'm enjoying life. This is my happiness window for body fat.

There's a science component to this as well. Below around 12–15% body fat we have lower leptin sensitivity and lower leptin levels meaning we're more likely to overeat, we'll struggle to gain muscle, but we will gain fat easily.

Conversely at about 25% body fat we have decreased fat oxidation (it's harder to burn fat, we have lower insulin sensitivity, and we can gain fat easily and struggle to gain muscle.).

So there is an optimum window...

Have a think about what yours might be.

A few years ago, in my mid-forties I had an amazing six-pack. Let me just tell you this, to get it took a huge amount of hard work. Of course, there was gym time, but getting there is often about really, really restricting your diet. I can tell you it's no fun at all. I thought I looked fantastic but actually people told me I looked ill and it turns out having a six pack didn't make me any happier, in fact it made me a bit sad because I was missing out on things that I enjoyed.

So I just tell that story to set realistic expectations for where you are now and what you think you might want...

Can you get to that goal? Of course you can. But it comes to what you're prepared to sacrifice to get there.

I suggest most of us would be happy losing a decent amount of weight, toning up our muscles and feeling that we look good without going to an extreme and starting to avoid entire food types, really monitoring what we're doing because you absolutely don't need to do that to get in the best shape of your life.

So where are you now? What's a realistic goal?

By the way, a lot of stuff you see out there isn't real, I'm in the fitness world, a lot of coaches out there will do this thing of getting into this kind of shape, but then get a photographer and take literally 1000s of photos, different locations, different outfits, and then put those out over time so it looks like they're in that shape permanently. They're not.

If you want to be in this kind of shape, you've got to make a ton of sacrifices and staying there will make you miserable. So there's trade offs and sacrifices and results. So just think, firstly, what's a great outcome for you? Because you can still achieve a great outcome for you without having to go through the massive sacrifices.

That's all part of this approach, no big sacrifices.

# If You Want, You Must...

*Results only work if you do, so here's what you've got to do once you're reading this book, because just reading it isn't enough – you need to take action on what's in it.*

If you were to go and talk to 100 different health coaches, there'll be approximately 936114 different things they'll tell you to do. Let me make it simple for you. I've trained thousands of clients, and I've discovered three main things that consistently deliver the results:

1. Align your body and mind
2. Commit and take action
3. Be consistent.

Those three things might not be sexy, but they sure as hell work.

Where people go wrong is making predictable mistakes, of which there are thousands. These mistakes are going to hold you back, keep you from having the body, health and happiness you desire and it's not your fault. You just don't know this stuff.

Here's some common myths, mistakes and misconceptions I see all the time:

- Dr. Google – trying to piece it all together by yourself with conflicting information.
- Doing more and more cardio for a longer period of time to lose body fat, it's not going to work, guys, it's not going to work, you're going to actually increase your stress response and cause your body to hold on to fat.

- Thinking activities like yoga or walking are enough. I get clients and I ask them, "What do you do for fitness?" "Oh, I do yoga once a week. So I'm really fit." No you're not. Yoga is great for breathing, for calming the mind. It helps with strength but flexibility is not a fitness activity. Some people may argue differently but in 10 years running retreats every single client (dozens) that said they just do yoga and they're fit, they really weren't when it came to training at anything else. I didn't have one case in all that time where someone that just did yoga could put in a good performance at HIIT, circuits, running, hill sprints...
- Doing things like skipping breakfast, or skipping meals as a way to cut calories. Or the other extreme eating whatever you want, as long as your calories are about on target
- Relying on supplements helps you lose weight. Most of them don't work and you don't need them
- Not eating enough of the right macros, or not getting your macros in the right ratios. My approach is not to overwhelm you with counting calories and measuring macros, but to give you an idea of what your plate should look like. So you can start intuitively tailoring your meals without stressing
- Ignoring the importance of your beliefs and self identity. You cannot outperform your self identity. So what's yours when it comes to your health, body, psychology?
- Ignoring the impact of stress. Stress has a massive impact on your physiologically, hormonally, emotionally, mentally
- Shrinking your calories too much – not eating enough basically
- Working against your midlife hormones, not really understanding what's happening inside under the bonnet so to speak. Understanding what you need to do to work in line with what's going on chemically for you, so you get the results you're after
- Not understanding the impact of sugar. Sugar is absolutely everything. Most of us consume far too much of it which has an inflammatory effect on the body and on the brain. It actually ages our brain and it's highly addictive. So we want to start cutting sugar down as much as we can

So there's where people go wrong. How about getting it right?

# Here's What We Need To Be Doing

*In the next chapter I'm going to give you some specific <u>Performance Principles</u> for different areas of your life, but before we drill down into the details let's review what we need to be doing to optimise our physical, mental and emotional health at midlife as men.*

Here's a summary of the ten areas we'll cover in more detail:

## Life Balance

Prioritising the Essential Areas:

In the hustle of everyday life, it's common for crucial aspects to receive less attention. Evaluate whether you're dedicating adequate time and energy to what truly matters. For instance, is your career overshadowing your relationships? Finding balance involves assessing and allocating time to relationships, career, health and personal growth to ensure a fulfilling life.

## Understanding Hormones

Insight into Changes:

When we have a clearer idea of what's driving the changes we're experiencing along with our feelings and behaviours we can adapt more effectively. These changes influence not only physical symptoms but also emotions and behaviours. Being aware of these shifts allows for better adaptation and management strategies, promoting emotional resilience during this phase.

## Nutrition

Comprehensive Diet Approach:

A well-rounded diet is pivotal during andropause. Focus on nutrient-dense foods, including lean proteins (chicken, fish, legumes), a vibrant variety of fruits and vegetables, whole grains, and healthy fats (avocado, nuts, olive oil). Ensure sufficient intake of calcium and vitamin D for maintaining bone health. Minimise processed foods, sugars, and excessive salt intake for optimal health benefits.

## Exercise

Holistic Physical Activity:

Regular exercise offers a multitude of benefits during andropause. Aim for a balanced routine encompassing aerobic exercises (walking, cycling, swimming) to enhance cardiovascular health, strength training (weightlifting, resistance exercises) for muscle maintenance, and flexibility exercises (stretching, yoga) to improve overall mobility and mood.

## Sleep

Prioritising Quality Rest:

Quality sleep plays a crucial role in hormone regulation and overall wellbeing during andropause. Establish a consistent sleep schedule, create a relaxing bedtime routine, and ensure a comfortable sleep environment. Minimise exposure to screens before bedtime and reduce stimulants like caffeine for better sleep quality.

## Stress Management

Strategies for Stress Reduction:

Chronic stress can exacerbate andropause symptoms. Employ stress-relief techniques such as deep breathing exercises, meditation, mindfulness, or yoga. Engage in activities that promote relaxation and reduce stress, fostering emotional wellbeing.

## Positive Mindset

Cultivating Positivity:

Actively work on developing a positive mindset. Recognise the impact of changing hormone levels on psychology and actively work towards cultivating a positive outlook. Practices like gratitude, affirmations, discipline and focusing on strengths contribute to a positive mindset.

## Avoidance Of Harmful Habits And Fostering Of Positive Ones

Change your Neural Pathways for Success:

When we form a habit we create a neural pathway and the more we practise that habit, the more robust that pathway becomes, making the habit easier and easier for us to do unconsciously. Think of brushing your teeth, you've done it thousands of times so you don't even think about it. Bearing that in mind we want to be aware of the habits that are taking us away from our goals and cultivate new habits that are going to help us become the person we want to be. For example you might decide to limit or avoid excessive alcohol consumption and quit smoking, because you know that substance abuse can disrupt hormonal balance and negatively impact overall health, worsening andropause symptoms. Start building healthier habits like moving your body regularly through the week.

## Social Connections, Values, Passion And Purpose

Nurturing Social Connections and Personal Fulfilment:

Loneliness kills more people than smoking. Fact. Men are worse at maintaining social networks than women. Fact. Maintain social connections and seek support from friends, family, or support groups. Social interactions can positively impact mental health, reduce feelings of isolation, and provide emotional support during challenging times. Reconnect with your values, your passions and decide on a purpose for your life to foster a sense of fulfilment and direction.

In addition, think about your goals – success is rarely achieved in isolation. Who do you need on your team to succeed? Who is in your trusted network? Who would you like to be?

Connecting with like-minded individuals will help you learn from others, widen your circle, create an environment where you can share ideas and find opportunities. It's also good to have mates!

## Supplements

Consideration for Additional Support:

Certain supplements have demonstrated efficacy in promoting hormonal health. Considering supplementation, in addition to a balanced diet, can provide necessary nutrients that might be lacking and contribute to improved overall health.

Implementing these lifestyle strategies can help men effectively manage symptoms associated with andropause while promoting overall health and wellbeing.

As a final note, you should also prioritise regular medical check-ups: schedule routine health check-ups with a healthcare provider. Regular monitoring of blood pressure, cholesterol levels, and hormone levels can help detect any underlying health issues and address them promptly.

# Your Performance Principles In Detail

## PERFORMANCE PRINCIPLE 1:
## 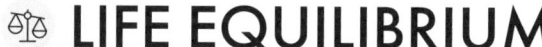 LIFE EQUILIBRIUM

Performance principle one is a short one, but it's arguably the most important, and it's about aligning the body and mind. I call this Life Equilibrium.

Like any route we might embark on, if we don't know where we're starting from, and we don't know where we're going, how are we ever going to arrive, let alone enjoy the journey?

Here's a little exercise I get my clients to do when they start working with me. We basically look at just four things: your body/health, work/finance, relationships and self. We look at where you are currently, that is how much energy or effort you're currently expanding on those and no surprise, most people are putting a lot into things like work and finance and tend not to be putting a lot into things like self-care. Sadly, relationships and body and health also tend to score low relative to career and finances.

We look at what the optimal energy expenditure in each area would be, that is where we would like to focus our energy.

Then we look at where the gap is. Once we've identified the gap (and it's often quite an eye opener), then we can start to set a goal from an energy perspective, and understand how we want to align our body and mind and spend our time.

Think of this as the foundation or keystone. We need to align and have a starting point and a target.

You'll find this Life Equilibrium as the first exercise in the Mindset section of the programme.

## CASE STUDY: **TIM (62)**

Tim is the CEO of a multinational company and he came to me feeling tired, lacking energy and focus and with a persistent shoulder injury that had gone on for years, impacting his ability to enjoy his hobby.

I addressed his physical challenges with an exercise programme that helped him drop excess body fat and build lean muscle, all while rehabilitating his shoulder injury. This included strength training, flexibility work, and mobility exercises. Over time, Tim regained strength in his shoulder and began to feel more physically capable.

In parallel, we revamped Tim's nutrition. His diet was already pretty good, but we made small tweaks that over time had a big impact, including ensuring sufficient protein. The changes in his diet not only fuelled his workouts but also gave him the mental clarity and sustained energy he needed to perform at his best in the office and beyond.

However, the real transformation came when we addressed Tim's mindset and lifestyle. He got to the point where he could delegate more effectively at work, empowering his leadership team while still driving the company's growth. By letting go of day-to-day control, Tim was able to step back and embrace a more strategic role, one that allowed him to focus on what mattered most to him both in and out of the office.

Within a few months, the changes in Tim's life were remarkable. Physically, he had dropped body fat, built lean muscle, got stronger and regained his energy. His shoulder injury, which had held him back for years, was no longer an issue and Tim was able to return to his hobby, taking it to the next level.

Tim also experienced a profound shift in his personal and professional life. By delegating effectively at work, he grew the company while simultaneously freeing up more time for himself. He learned to step into a leadership role that didn't require him to be involved in every detail, giving him more space to focus on strategic decisions and long-term vision giving him a newfound freedom.

# PERFORMANCE PRINCIPLE 2:
# ⚥ UNDERSTANDING HORMONES

This one is massive, we need to understand our midlife male hormones. Specifically we need to understand how they are impacting not just our body but our mood and mind as well.

As men, from about 40 onwards (it will vary from individual to individual), we're all going through something called andropause.

Think of andropause as age-related testosterone decline. For men our testosterone levels peak in our 20s and then decline at a steady rate of 1 to 2% per year, which doesn't sound a lot but when you're compounding it, you can see by the time you're in your 50s you could have testosterone levels somewhere between 30–50% lower than they were when you were in your 20s.

You're probably familiar with some facts about testosterone, but there's also a lot of misconception about it. Testosterone is not just about libido, muscle and energy, but is responsible for a whole host of functions in the body and brain. Here are some facts about it:

1. Testosterone is an essential hormone in both men and women.
2. Declining testosterone IS associated with healthy ageing BUT low levels are not and can cause a significant reduction in quality of life.
3. Testosterone fluctuates in males over a 24 hour period and is highest in the mornings.
4. 40% of men over 45 have low levels of testosterone.
5. 9 out of 10 men never seek help as they think it's normal to feel lethargic, achy and less youthful.
6. Low levels can cause weight gain, loss of muscle mass, lowered self confidence, low libido, insomnia, erectile dysfunction and brain fog.
7. Optimal levels strengthen bones, increase red blood cell production and keep muscles strong as well as increasing energy levels, cognitive function and sex drive.
8. Testosterone plays a role in cognition and brain function.
9. Prolonged stress can further depress your natural testosterone levels.
10. Testosterone replacement therapy can be an option, but won't really work unless we also dial in the lifestyle factors we're covering here.

Now, testosterone plays a role obviously in libido, in energy, it plays a role in metabolism, it plays a role in our muscle mass. So when our testosterone is declining, we can put on belly fat, we can lose motivation and confidence, we can lose our libido, we can suffer from erectile dysfunction, and a load of other symptoms that we really ideally don't want.

Here is a big list of symptoms:

- loss of muscle mass and strength
- decreased bone density
- lowered metabolism
- increased body fat, particularly in the abdominal area
- decreased energy levels
- loss of libido
- depression
- anxiety
- nocturia (which means increased need to urinate at night)
- insomnia
- reducing head and body hair
- decreased motivation
- decreased confidence
- brain fog
- increased stress

This is not an exhaustive list, but these are really common guys. Can you relate? I'm sure you can. And most of these are driven by that fall in testosterone.

But it's not just testosterone. Many other hormones and neurotransmitters are in a state of flux and I refer to this as the "portfolio effect" as these changes can actually amplify negative symptoms as well.

For example, as we age we have increased insulin resistance which basically means we're less efficient at processing the food we eat for energy and are more likely to store the excess energy as fat. We have decreasing levels of the hormone leptin, our satiety hormone, so we're more likely to overeat.

So why is it important? Well, testosterone plays a role for our skin, in our muscles, in our bones, our sex organs, our bone marrow, our brain, it does so much in our body. And when we start to go low on it, obviously, we're going to start to feel the effects of it.

Levels of human growth hormone are in decline, which plays a role in an overall healthy body building new tissue, ensuring regular sleep cycles, and helps regulate your body composition and metabolism, meaning we're more likely to put on body fat.

If we're stressed (and we'll cover this in a moment) then stress hormone cortisol is going to amplify all of the above negative effects.

Finally our neurotransmitters which govern mood and cognition can also be disrupted, with lower levels of feel good hormone serotonin in particular having an impact.

So with all these changes going on, it's no surprise that they can in turn drive psychological impacts as well. If we are low on energy, anxious, putting on weight, our libido is low, then that in turn can drive negative thought patterns and create a kind of negative feedback loop.

The good news is that knowing all of this, there are 100% steps we can take to work in line with all these changes to alleviate these symptoms and bring us back to an even keel.

So here's a quick word on testosterone replacement therapy. Now, everything else I'm going to show you in this book is about the natural approach. It's about lifestyle techniques, and tweaks that you can make to actually work in line with your hormones and build a better outcome for yourself and optimise your performance.

However, if your testosterone levels are already low, you might want to see your health professional to get a blood test for testosterone levels. Then you can decide whether testosterone replacement therapy is an option for you. But even if you do go down that road, it is not a miracle cure, you cannot just start taking TRT and still carry on not exercising, eating junk food, not looking after your mindset, you have to do all the stuff I'm going to share with you now as well.

I'm aware I've painted a negative picture here, but awareness gives us the power to make educated adjustments. It's good to know what's happening rather than being in the dark and chalking it up to age, or stress, or a bad month at work. Knowing what's going on means you can take steps to do something about it. You're not alone, it's not your fault.

That ends now.

# PERFORMANCE PRINCIPLE 3:
# 🍎 NUTRITION

You can't out perform a bad diet and this becomes even more true as we age. Truth bomb – constant dieting is making you fat! Yes really.

If diet books worked there wouldn't be a new one every month! The problem is we live in a quick fix society, and it's all about how much can I lose (weight wise) and how quickly. I get it, but you didn't put all that weight on overnight, so why expect to lose it that way.

The truth is that dieting will wreck your body and your relationship with food, for no long term results. A bad relationship with food not only keeps you locked in a vicious and obsessive cycle, but fad diets will ruin your body from the inside out. I see this time and time again, people who've done diet after diet after diet… it takes so long to reset their metabolism back to the point where it's running effectively, because the body just doesn't know what's going on.

Instead we want to get to a point where we can make good choices, where we can enjoy beers and not worry about it. No sacrifices, just balance.

Where we go wrong, we turn to things like shake plans, or cutting this food group or fasting for these days or taking these supplements… sure all these things can get results in the short term but they're not fixing the root of the problem. They're not educating you on how you should be nourishing yourself.

The root of the word nutrition is nourishment. Fad diets only work for the short term, they make you miserable and set you back to where you started. Or worse, here's a stat: 97% of dieters put on the same weight or more within three years of finishing their diet. I'd say that's a conservative estimate and a long period of time. In my experience most people have regained the weight they lost (and then some) in 6 months or less. Diets just DO NOT work guys.

> *"Instead we want to get to a point where we can make good choices, where we can enjoy beers and not worry about it. No sacrifices, just balance."*

You end up in a yo-yo cycle that crashes your metabolism, you get locked into this vicious cycle. You're restricting yourself all the time, you start thinking about all the things you can't have and start getting miserable. If I say to you that you can't eat chocolate cake what's the first thing you want? It's no way to be living and it's not a healthy way to do it.

Also, you're depriving your body of essential nutrients, which is bad news, because you're already losing your muscles and your bone density. On top of that you get locked into bad habits and you start to blame yourself for your long term lack of success. I'm sure you can relate to that.

But here's the good news, there is a way you can have it all, within reason, of course, but it is possible. I love a burger, pizza, beer... so do lots of people that work with me, and that's not a problem. The difference comes in making good choices 80% of the time and having what you want the other 20%. That cuts the feeling of restriction, and you still get results.

The idea is to simplify nutrition. You don't need another diet, you just need good nutritional principles to guide you.

A bad relationship with food and not understanding it keeps you locked in a vicious and obsessive cycle and diet fads (& feast & famine!) will ruin your midlife body – from the inside out.

The yo-yo dieting crashes your metabolism and keeps you locked in a miserable cycle that lowers your self confidence, self esteem and indeed your immune system.

You feel trapped in bad habits – as you never really understand how or why your diets DON'T work – and blame yourself.

There is a way to have it all – dare I say it... to have your cake and eat it!

And real results that last are only achieved when you're educated and empowered.

No more hunger. No more sacrifices...

Here's the problem: we're never taught this stuff so we don't know how to make good choices. Broadly speaking our food can be split into one of three macro groups: protein, fats and carbohydrates.

Most of us are eating far too many carbohydrates, and too many processed and refined carbs. Carbohydrates are things like cake, bread, pasta, pastry, rice, potatoes, vegetables.

Ideally our carbs want to make up between 40–50% of our daily intake and we want those carbs to be mainly vegetables. We also want to load our carbohydrates early in the day, since if we load with carbs at night, all that energy isn't being utilised so is more likely to be stored as body fat.

So we want to start the day with a meal rich in carbs and protein, something like oats with protein powder, eggs on sourdough, a smoothie with a small amount of fruit, oats and protein.

We know that as we age we're becoming more insulin resistant, so we want to control our insulin response as much as possible. We can do that by minimising sugar in our diet, and when we do have it combine it with protein and/or fats to slow the release.

When we've fasted overnight we should wake up burning fat for energy, and what we first eat will set our insulin bandwidth for the day, so we do not want to be starting the day with anything sweet that's going to spike our insulin.

So sugary cereals are out, as are jams, chocolate spreads and normal bread (high in sugar) in favour of slow release energy foods like oats, eggs or a smoothie.

Have carbs with lunch and then a small amount of carbs in the evening. So we may have something like rice or a small amount of potatoes for lunch, and in the evening have mainly leafy greens, so a stir fry or oven roasted broccoli and asparagus.

Next up we have protein. Now we need more protein as we age to help build our muscle tissue (which we're losing), because our guts are less efficient at extracting protein from our food, and to trigger our leptin so we're less likely to overeat.

Protein can come from fish, poultry, lean red meats, nuts and pulses and we should be aiming for around one gram of protein per kilo of bodyweight as a minimum. If you're struggling to get this in then protein powders are a convenient way to boost your protein levels. You can add a scoop to water, to oats, to yogurt, to shakes – it's a great way to easily increase your protein intake.

Finally we have fats. Now we do need fat in our diet, particularly for our hormonal health. Again many of us have too many of the wrong kinds of fats, saturated fats (which come from meat and dairy products) – we need some, but we should be focusing on increasing our unsaturated fats which come from oily fish, nuts and seeds. The key fat we want to be getting is omega 3 as this plays a role in metabolism and hormone health. Aim for about 15–20% of your daily intake to be fats, mainly unsaturated.

So, in summary, 40–50% carbohydrates, 15–20% fats and 30–40% protein.

That's the macros. As previously stated we want to cut right back on processed and ultra processed foods as they impact our gut health (lowering mood), make us more likely to overeat, and lead to weight gain, as well as overriding our normal hormonal responses to food and being inflammatory to our body and brain.

A cautionary word here, these are guiding principles to simplify nutrition and with the aim of helping you drop body fat, increase lean muscle, have more energy and optimise your hormone health. These principles will work for the majority of people, if you want to take it to the next level, then of course, working with a nutritional therapist or similar, with multiple tests, monitoring and coaching could get you better results. But for bespoke, you of course, pay for the service. Start with these principles and if you're inspired down the line to learn more about nutrition, then by all means go down the bespoke route, just don't overcomplicate it at the start. The principles outlined here and in the 30-day programme will work in terms of making a positive impact to your overall wellbeing.

So, here's some action points. Make a note of these – small steps, big changes:

## Focus On Whole Foods And Cut Out All Processed Carbs.

So our body hormonally does not recognise ultra processed foods, things that have got lots of chemicals in it that have gone through many processes. Think things like "potato" chips in tubes that are actually full of chemicals, fake meat and many baked goods... Our body hormonally just doesn't recognise them. When we eat there are a number of hormonal processes that go on to help us digest and utilise food for energy. Ultra processed food overrides all of those and the research shows that given a diet equal in calories to a natural whole food diet, a diet high in UPFs (ultra processed foods) will result in more weight gain. The research also shows that if you take that calorie rule away, then you will consume in the region of 20–30% more calories when eating diets high in UPFs, so a double whammy. Not to mention chemicals, inflammation, low energy from poor nutrients...

## Cut Back Sugar

Now sugar is in everything – food manufacturers know that it's highly addictive, and that when we eat it we instantly crave more. NHS guidelines state that anything that is 21.5% sugar is a high sugar product, while anything 5% or lower is low sugar. You want to start checking your food labelling and you're looking for the "Carbohydrates: Of Which Sugars" label. This is telling you your sugar percentage. For years we've tended to prioritise low fat foods (based on flawed research from the 1980s that blamed fat for heart diseases and obesity) when the evidence suggests sugar is much more harmful. Be aware that when the fat is removed from food so is the flavour, so often lower fat versions will have far higher sugar content than the "regular" version. Most of our food is packed with hidden sugars. Sugar is highly calorific, highly addictive and when we eat it we get an insulin spike. The more we spike our insulin through consuming sugar the more insulin resistant we become and remember we're becoming more insulin resistant as we age anyway. Insulin resistance means we're more likely to store energy as fat, and left unchecked can lead to serious disease, like Type 2 Diabetes. So we want to bring sugar down and help train ourselves to become more insulin sensitive via our diet. Tip: a massive culprit for hidden sugars are "health" bars often with images of rabbits and animals on. In fact these bars rely on dried fruit and things like date sugar to bind them and their sugar content tends to be through the roof – so beware! Start checking your food labels – you'll be surprised...

## Don't Eat Your Carbs After 4pm

Front load them in the day. Groups given the same amount of calories and carbs but front loading them versus back loading them in the day (having them late in the day), result in the back loading groups putting on more weight. Which makes sense if you think about it, if we're onboarding with energy late in the day when we're less active, it's not utilised and so will be stored as fat. If you flip this on its head, this is why endurance athletes eat big carb heavy meals the night before an event, so they have more energy, but that is not what we want for our everyday lives. Basically most of us live the wrong way round, we have breakfast on the go, lunch on the go, then a big evening meal because that's how we set ourselves up. It's the wrong way round, instead you want to be doing breakfast like a king, lunch like a prince, dinner like a pauper. I want to be clear here that we're not saying go carb free, in fact we're totally not a low carb approach. We don't like keto as carbohydrates are the body's preferred energy source. The problem is too many of us are just eating too many of the wrong kind of carbs too late in the day. As an easy rule of thumb, avoid the beige and white; pasta, potatoes, rice, things like that, and instead go for lots of leafy greens, all the fresh colourful stuff that grows mainly above ground and eat them all earlier in the day. As a guide make sure that carbohydrates aren't more than 45% of your overall diet.

## Increase Your Lean Protein And Healthy Fats

Because they trigger a hormone called leptin, which is also in decline at this stage of life. Leptin is our satiety hormone. It's the "I'm full" hormone. Protein and healthy fats trigger it making you feel fuller for longer.

## Watch Your Portion Sizes And Know Your Go-To Snacks

This is where so many people go wrong. The overall food can be great, but it's the biscuits, chocolate, and sweets that they forget to "count" as part of their daily intake. Here's a tip, a lot of the time I start working with clients I get them to keep a food diary just for a little while, not just so I can see where they're at, but so they're more aware of where the extras might be slipping in. Sometimes there are no little extras and their diet could be really healthy, but they're just eating far too much. So know your portion sizes.

No one wants to be counting calories or weighing and measuring food, so a really cool way we teach people using your hand sizes is something you can start to use intuitively to then programme your food. This guide is in the Programme section of this book along with nutritional guidelines to get you started for 30-days.

So now you know your portion sizes, know your go-to snacks so when you're getting hungry rather than reaching for the biscuits or the crisps, know what else you can go to that's going to make you feel full straight away. Things like a teaspoon of good quality nut butter, a protein shake, cottage cheese, a small handful of raw nuts... all things that will trigger your leptin and are low in sugar.

## Start Thinking About Your Food Intake Over A Few Days Rather Than Daily

What I mean by that is if you know you have an event coming up where you'll overeat (or drink) then the day before and day after taper your consumption down, so that over a 2 to 3 day period the amount you eat equalises out. Remember, one big blow out meal is not going to make a difference, it's only if you keep doing it that it does. Achieving balance with your food is so empowering.

## Drink More Water

One great way to instantly have more energy is to drink more water. Most of us spend our days mildly dehydrated. When we're dehydrated we'll often confuse that for fatigue or hunger. Get into the practice of drinking a large glass of water as soon as you wake up, then aim for a minimum of two litres of water a day, more if you're exercising or sweating. I personally aim for around three litres a day. I've found that this stabilises my energy levels through the day so I no longer need caffeine as a pick up.

## Minimise Phyto-estrogens In Your Diet

Along with toxins and endocrine disrupting foods, Phyto-estrogens are foods that mimic female sex hormone oestrogen in the body. Needless to say as a man we want to be minimising the intake of these foods as much as possible. Various seeds contain them, but these also have benefits in terms of saturated fats and if you're eating them in small amounts then there's not an issue, but soya is a big culprit so this means avoiding soya and soy based products as much as possible (phyto-estrogen). Avoid BPA plastic containers for food and try and eat organic where possible to avoid exposure to pesticides, and additives in the food chain. Also avoid seed oils and beware of certain cosmetic products. Essentially we're looking to minimise toxins in our endocrine system.

## Eat Enough Fibre

If you're doing all the above then your gut health should improve, but do make sure you're eating enough natural fibres from vegetables and fruit to nourish your gut biomes, and regularly add in food with live cultures like live bio yoghurts and fermented foods. Our gut health plays a role in metabolism and mood, so boosting gut health has both physical and psychological benefits.

## Finally, Alcohol

Alcohol is antagonistic to our testosterone health. When we drink we have disturbed sleep, our recovery and in particular muscular recovery is impaired and our testosterone levels may dip. Aim to moderate your drinking or have spells where you don't drink at all.

That's it, simple principles.

Simplifying nutrition (and eliminating confusion) empowers you to take charge of your health for life AND builds positive habits.

Get it wrong and you'll create huge problems for yourself – bones, muscles, immune system.

Get it right and you're free from the obsessive, tortuous cycle of dieting and restrictions for good....

# PERFORMANCE PRINCIPLE 4: ⚡ UNDERSTANDING AND MANAGING STRESS

Understanding the science of stress and how it impacts you AND your hormones is key. Now there are thousands of books out there about stress, so we're not going to deep dive into it here, but we are going to cover why it matters, and give you some pointers on how to handle it so that you lessen its impact.

I'm sure you'll agree that we live in an increasingly stressful world. I'm not going to go through it all here, but these are just some of the things that can place stress on us...

We have careers, we have families, we have kids, we have ageing parents. We're trying to look after our own health. With so many things going on, it's hardly surprising that at times we can feel that the stress on us can be almost unbearable.

Before we get onto the negative side of stress, let's remember, stress isn't always bad. Stress is the body's way of protecting us, and it can help us rise to challenges. The problem comes when it's prolonged.

With stress we have a bell curve of performance, known as the Yerkes-Dodson Law, and ideally when we're focused on a task we want to reach that point of peak performance right at the top of the curve. Too little and we're not feeling the pressure enough to get that really great edge from our performance, too much and we're starting to degrade our performance as the stress becomes too much. Note that this curve is going to be different for every individual, and vary according to the stress or task as well. What gets one person stressed may not phase another and vice versa. The problem comes when we're at the peak for too long as we can't stay in that peak performance window, we will burn out. So we want to be operating somewhere in that optimum stress zone, coming up and going down and coming up and going down.

## The Yerkes-Dodson Stress Curve

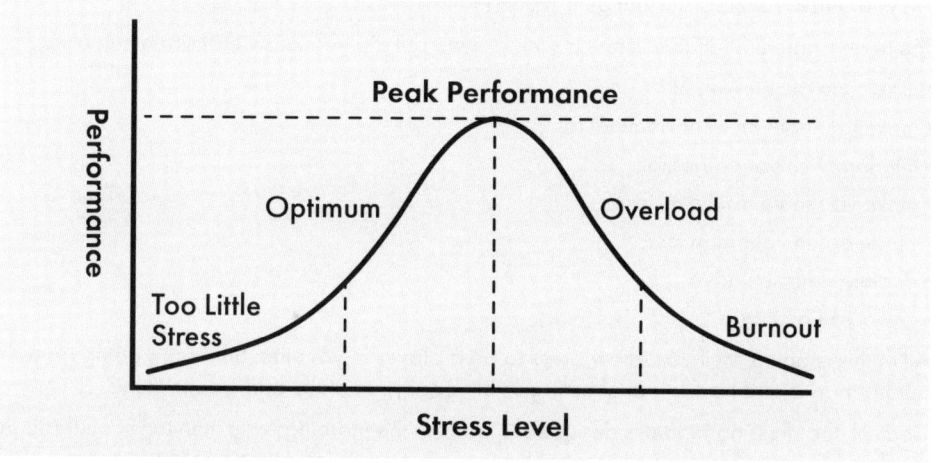

What tends to happen in life though is that we get overloaded, not necessarily by one thing but by a combination of stressors, so that over time we slip over the peak of the curve and we start to lose our effectiveness. If we don't do anything to address it, then eventually we'll burn out and break down.

So stress isn't all bad, it does have a function in helping us reach our peak performance, but in the context of health on a day to day basis we want to be looking at ways of reducing our stress so it's not impacting us or our hormones.

Because here's the thing, consistent stress is incredibly bad for us. It's a silent killer.

In modern life we've become used to living with a constant background hum of stress. We live in an 'always on' society where we gauge our value by what we're achieving and we've become human 'doings' instead of human beings. It's just not good for us.

Most of us believe that success is based on what we have rather than what we are, we're always chasing the next thing to be happy. We've become used to the expectations placed on us from society and we don't take the time to sit still and create space. We fail to set boundaries. Compounding that, we increasingly have this lack of human to human connection.

It's fair to say that we still have a stigma around stress, there's still an element of shame and guilt admitting we're stressed and can't cope — instead sometimes we wear it like a badge of honour... "Oh, I'm so stressed."

We're getting confused between the difference between busy-ness and stress. Or when we're really stressed and it's making us ill or it's impairing performance, we almost don't want to admit it, there's still that guilt around it.

The health impact of chronic stress is well known, but did you know that stress can also:

- make you put on weight
- make you hold on to abdominal fat
- interfere with your digestion
- make you more insulin resistant
- break down your muscles
- deplete your sex drive
- make you anxious

All of this is going on if you allow stress to be a player in your life. So what's going on with our hormones and how is that affecting us physically, mentally and emotionally?

Cortisol, the stress hormone, is designed to peak in the mornings and then taper off through the day. However for many of us what happens is it peaks and then just keeps going.

That's bad news. Remember that stress is a flight or fight survival mechanism so our body preps for physical exertion that doesn't come. Our heart rate and blood pressure go up, our blood sugar increases, blood moves away from our internal organs to our muscles and our pain sensitivity decreases.

All great if we are in an actual physical conflict, not so great for a day in the office, or while trying to chill out with the family.

The stress chemical cocktail essentially shuts down any non combat/running essential processes: like digestion (IBS anyone?) and libido (yep stress can take away your desire). At the same time your brain focuses on the perceived stressor at the expense of the wider environment leading to brain fog or confusion — remember this is already happening thanks to declining testosterone (and other hormones) so stress is amplifying it.

As our blood sugar rises and stays elevated over time we start to lose insulin sensitivity, just as we're becoming more insulin resistant anyway.

Then there's the effect of raised cortisol itself, it encourages the body to lay down fat, particularly in the abdominal area. See how various processes in the body are combining to actually work against what you want to achieve? The good news is that understanding this means we can take steps to remedy it.

Here's another effect, serotonin production decreases. Now serotonin is mainly made in the gut. It's our feel good happy hormone. So when we're stressed, we start to feel more anxious and depressed.

I'd like to draw your attention to the stress hormone pathway diagram below, because I think it really helps to understand what's going on the next time you are getting stressed.

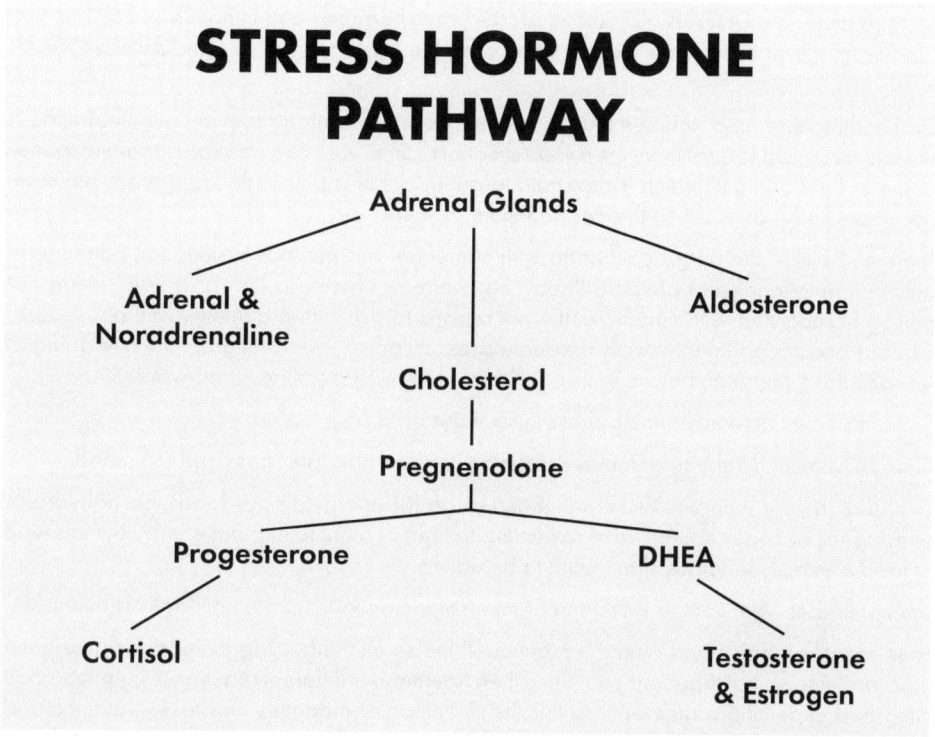

I want to draw your attention to the two branches coming down at the bottom of the tree and you'll see at the bottom of one of the legs is cortisol, the stress hormone. If you go up the leg to where it branches, you'll see what we call the mother hormone pregnenolone.

Now pregnenolone is responsible for making another hormone called DHEA, which in turn makes our sex hormones – so our testosterone and a little bit of oestrogen for us guys. What's interesting is if we're allowing that stress to be a constant player in our life, if it's that constant hum and we're producing cortisol, there's less pregnenolone available to make the DHEA, which means less testosterone.

Cortisol is like the alpha male hormone, it overrides the others, taking top priority and taking resources away from them, so that stress is actually stealing our testosterone away. Stress is stealing your testosterone. Which is why when you're stressed, you can get low on energy, your libido can go, this is all the effects of your testosterone being taken away.

On a related note DHEA is also known as the youth hormone and if there's less of that, you age faster – ever seen someone that's had a big trauma and they've aged quickly? Here's why.

So if nothing else, bear this in mind, you have to learn to control stress in your life. Because stress is supposed to exist there for a short amount of time, we have an evolutionary response to stress 'fight or flight' which is designed to get us out of a physically dangerous situation, but instead most of us live in this constant hum of stress.

The email pings, the angry exchange with someone, our nervous system can't distinguish between emotional and physical threat. So, we're not facing a lion or a tiger, we're just getting bombarded with emails, with work reports to do, with arguments with our spouse, and our body is going to exactly the same stress response, which is great if we're going to do something physical, but we're not. So it's causing disease, illness and worse.

So here's how I advise handling stress in six ways:

One, movement. Make sure you're exercising. It helps alleviate stress and lifts mood.

Two, dial in your nutrition. Stress will make us go for energy, heavy foods, carbohydrates and sugars, because again, we're expecting to fight or flight to expend energy but this type of food is exactly what we don't want to be eating.

Three, mindset. We want to work on our mindset to become more emotionally resilient.

Four, identify triggers and work on reaction. If the same thing is triggering you figure out if you can remove that trigger. If you can't, then figure out a different reaction. Doing the same thing and expecting a different result is the definition of madness. This takes patience and awareness but is possible and will pay dividends in reducing your stress levels over time.

Five, environment. We want to ensure that we're in as much of a stress free environment as we can make it. So how's your space at home? Your work space? What can you do to declutter them, to make them more comfortable? Watch what you're feeding yourself... are you watching too much news? Is your social media stream stressing you out? You're in control of these things. Clean your feed, turn off the TV.

*"Remember, it's not the stress that kills us. It's our reaction to it."*

Six, spirituality. Having a greater connection to yourself or to something bigger. There's a lot of research from the field of positive psychology that shows when we are feeling more connected to ourselves or to a higher purpose, our stress levels decline so we can feel more of our place in the universe.

Remember, it's not the stress that kills us. It's our reaction to it.

# PERFORMANCE PRINCIPLE 5: THE POWER OF EXERCISE

Performance principle four is movement, aka exercise. Ageing is a natural process, but we can offset the effects, which is great news, right?

Exercise is good for us in a multitude of ways: physically, mental and emotionally – Public Health guidelines for the UK tell us we should:

Be active at moderate intensity for 150 minutes per week

OR

75 minutes intense activity per week

OR a combination of the two

PLUS at least 2 strength training sessions a week

QUESTION: Be honest with yourself, how much movement is your body really getting at the moment?

We've covered hormones, so you can see that one of the effects we face is that we're basically losing muscle mass, we're losing our strength and losing our physique. Muscle is metabolically active so as we lose it our metabolism slows down and we're more likely to put on weight as fat. We also lose bone density putting us at risk of osteoporosis and fractures, frailty and falls. No one wants that and it doesn't have to be like this.

Here are some health benefits of exercise:
- Improves sleep
- Lowers stress
- Maintains healthy weight
- Improves quality of life
- Improves mood
- Lowers anxiety

Reduces the risk of:
- Type 2 Diabetes by 40%
- Cardiovascular disease by 35%
- Risk of falls 30%
- Joint and back pain 25%
- Cancers 20%
- Lower all risk mortality!
- It makes you feel good, look good, gives you confidence and improves almost all areas of your life

It really is a case of use or lose it as we age, but we need to apply science. We can't train like we might have done in our 20s or 30s. We're hormonally and physiologically very different. We need to train for shorter periods in specific ways with adequate recovery time around those training periods. The ideal way to achieve this, hit your goals, maintain them and feel great is by combining resistance training alongside cardio.

Broadly exercise can be split into cardio/aerobic and resistance type training.

Of course some types of training (cross fit, circuits with equipment) are both.

## Cardio 101

The word cardio can be off putting for some. We get that. But put simply, all we mean is elevating your heart rate so that you increase your fitness, raise your metabolic rate and burn through calories and fat more efficiently.

The benefits of this are life longevity, more energy, a lifted mood and of course a change in your physique.

You can do your cardio in a wide variety of ways with differing levels of intensity

Here are some types of cardio:

## Low Intensity Steady State (LISS)
- Walking
- Swimming
- Slow jog
- Gentle cycle

## Moderate Intensity Steady State (MISS)
- Running
- Cycling
- Crosstrainer
- Rowing

## High Intensity Interval Training (HIIT)
- Circuits
- Sprints

Ideally mix up all of these approaches, however if you are time poor then a good approach is 2 x HIIT plus a MISS or LISS per week.

HIIT is the methodology we know works the quickest in the least amount of time. We've used it with clients for years and it's the main form of cardio that keeps our bodies in shape – while still enjoying the finer things in life!

You only need 15 to 20 minutes of HIIT and your other session can be 30 to 120 minutes.

Research has shown that HIIT is one of the few methodologies that can actually reduce biological age when you look at markers like inflammation in the body. So regular HIIT sessions actually bring your biological age down, if you have adequate recovery times.

HIIT also creates an oxygen debt, meaning we speed up the metabolism for the next 24 to 48 hours, meaning we're burning more calories, so it helps manage our fat levels. It also releases endorphins, we get an endorphin rush making us feel good. And here's the thing, when we're doing HIIT consistently, even on the days we don't do it, we'll start to produce those endorphins.

Finally intense cardio elicits a hormonal response temporarily elevating levels of testosterone and human growth hormone.

## Cardio Hints And Tips

- If fat loss or weight management is your goal you can do HIIT fasted – early in the morning – either at the gym or at home, your body will burn through residual glucose and glycogen and turn to body fat for energy

- Remember to eat straight after your cardio workout if you can – a protein based meal with simple carbs as this helps bring cortisol down as we want to keep workout stress low

- Sip your water! Don't gulp it during cardio sessions – it'll give you a stitch! But do make sure you drink plenty each day – at least 2 litres please

- Wear decent trainers for your cardio – they'll protect your knees

- You do not need to go to the gym to do your cardio – so there really are no excuses! Lots of our clients do this at home, even while travelling in hotel rooms!

## Resistance (Weights) 101

Resistance or strength training are going to SHAPE you and make you STRONG. It's essential to do both HIIT and Resistance because we not only want to lower body fat (or keep it stable), but also build muscle.

Muscle not only makes you look leaner (and better naked!), but when you have muscle, you're burning more fat. Muscle takes more energy to repair and therefore we burn more calories at rest (in fact 1lbs of fat burns around 2 calories per day and 1lbs of muscle can burn up to 50 calories a day!).

You need to work each muscle group at least twice a week to get results but you should never work the same muscle group within 48 hours as this is when the tissue is repairing.

This could mean two longer full body sessions per week OR

You can split your workouts to suit your lifestyle e.g. Push/Pull, Upper/Lower and do 3 to 4 shorter workouts each week.

You can resistance train at home using your bodyweight, or use simple equipment like bands and kettlebells.

Of course the other option is the gym where you have both free weights and machines.

With resistance training we work in sets of reps for example 3 sets of 10 reps with rest in between the sets.

In terms of set up you should be looking to work your muscle close to failure – so this could mean high reps with a lower weight or lower reps with a high weight.

A basic rule of thumb is:

- Strength = high number of sets, low reps, high weight e.g. 10 sets of 5 reps, long rests 3 to 4 minutes

- Endurance (the ability to maintain a prolonged effort) = low number of sets, high reps, low weight e.g. 2 sets of 25 reps, short rests 30 seconds

- Hypertrophy (muscular size) = medium number of sets, medium number of reps, medium weight e.g. 3 sets of 12 reps, medium rests 1 minute

Nothing is more important than your safety and good form so if you're unsure always ask a trainer to guide you.

Lifting weights and particularly compound movements that work multiple muscle groups (think squat, deadlift, row, press…) give a temporary boost to testosterone and human growth hormone.

This means that regular sessions are going to help maintain optimised hormone levels, as well as giving us those feel good neurotransmitters.

A word on DOMS (Delayed Onset Muscle Stress) is normal – which means you will be sore if you're not used to doing weights/resistance training.

## **Resistance Hints And Tips**

- Start lighter and aim to increase your reps and or weight over time

- Change your programme every 8 weeks or so as your body adapts

- Make sure you're getting enough protein in to help build muscle

- Ensure you work each muscle group twice a week with at least 48 hours between workouts for the same body part

- If you're sore – try taking a magnesium supplement or using a magnesium oil spray. Why magnesium? Because it's necessary for proper muscle function. It works with other essential minerals in your body to keep the muscles loose and flexible

# PERFORMANCE PRINCIPLE 6: SLEEP AND RECOVERY

Adequate and quality sleep is fundamental for maintaining hormonal balance, including optimising testosterone levels. This is because testosterone production occurs predominantly during sleep, specifically during the rapid eye movement (REM) stage which is one of the deepest stages of sleep. So if our sleep is disturbed or too short, then our testosterone is going to be impacted.

## The Impact Of Sleep Deprivation On Testosterone Levels

Chronic sleep deprivation or poor sleep quality can negatively impact testosterone production and regulation. Studies have shown that inadequate sleep, irregular sleep patterns, or disrupted sleep can lead to reduced testosterone levels. Sleep disturbances alter the endocrine system, impacting the hypothalamic-pituitary-gonadal axis, which regulates testosterone production, leading to potential hormonal imbalances.

Ideally you want to be aiming for 8 hours of quality sleep a night.

Sleep quality also affects cortisol levels, a stress hormone that influences testosterone levels. Elevated cortisol levels due to insufficient or poor-quality sleep can suppress testosterone production. High stress levels negatively impact the production and regulation of hormones, including testosterone, thereby affecting overall hormonal balance.

We call this the sleep/stress cycle. We're stressed, so we sleep poorly, meaning we're more stressed, so we sleep poorly.... And of course it works the other way too – you'll know how frazzled you can feel after a poor night's sleep.

## Optimal Sleep And Recovery Practices

To optimise testosterone health and overall hormonal balance during midlife, prioritise the following sleep and recovery practices:

Consistent Sleep Schedule: Maintain a regular sleep routine by going to bed and waking up at the same time every day, even on weekends, to support the body's natural circadian rhythm.

Create a Sleep-Conducive Environment: Ensure a comfortable sleep environment that is dark, quiet, and cool to promote uninterrupted sleep.

Limit Stimulants: Reduce or avoid stimulants like caffeine, particularly close to bedtime, to improve sleep quality.

Manage Stress: Engage in stress-reduction techniques such as meditation, deep breathing exercises, or relaxation practices to minimise cortisol levels and promote better sleep.

Limit Screen Time: Minimise exposure to electronic devices before bedtime as blue light emitted from screens can disrupt the body's natural production of melatonin, a hormone essential for sleep regulation.

Regular Exercise: Incorporate regular physical activity into your routine, but avoid vigorous exercise close to bedtime, as it may interfere with sleep.

If you're really struggling with sleep, then sleeping pills are a plaster. Instead seek guidance from healthcare professionals, such as sleep specialists, who can provide personalised recommendations and interventions tailored to individual needs.

In summary, prioritising adequate and quality sleep, along with incorporating effective recovery practices, is crucial for optimising testosterone health and overall hormonal balance during midlife. Implementing these strategies contributes not only to better sleep but also supports hormonal regulation, vitality, and overall wellbeing.

# PERFORMANCE PRINCIPLE 7: TRANSFORMING HABITS

Along with your beliefs, your habits are what are going to inform your success or failure when it comes to making lifestyle changes. Indeed it could be said that humans are nothing more than a bundle of beliefs and habits, they're so strong that they run unconsciously and inform many aspects of our behaviour.

Of course that's great if the habits are working for us, but if they're not then we need to do some work. Now changing habits isn't easy, but it's a lot easier than sticking with habits that will derail you. The good news is that it is possible to change habits. You're going to have to work at it consciously, but over time, the more you practise, the more the neural pathways form, the more unconscious it will become over time. We'll look at brain plasticity in more detail later, but in essence you can imagine neural pathways as the roads in our brain which the electrical impulses, that are our thoughts, travel down.

Remember when you learned to drive a car? The first time you sat behind the wheel it probably felt overwhelming – gears, a wheel, indicators, mirrors and you're moving fast!

But if you've learnt to drive you'll know that now you can drive without even thinking about it. This is what we want to achieve when creating new habits for our success.

Here's how:

## 1. Identify Specific Habits For Change

Identifying specific habits involves self-reflection and pinpointing behaviours that negatively impact health or hormonal balance. These could include excessive alcohol consumption, smoking, poor dietary choices, sedentary lifestyles, irregular sleep patterns, or high-stress levels. Understanding which habits to alter is the initial step towards positive change. Aim to work on only two to three habits maximum at a time.

## 2. Set Clear And Achievable Goals

Establishing clear and achievable goals provides direction and motivation for habit change. Define specific, measurable, attainable, relevant, and time-bound (SMART) objectives. For instance, set a goal to reduce alcohol intake by a certain percentage within a defined time frame or commit to exercising a certain number of days per week.

## 3. Understand The "Why"

Understanding the reasons behind changing habits adds purpose and motivation. Reflect on the benefits of altering these behaviours—how it contributes to better health, enhanced wellbeing, increased energy levels, and optimised testosterone. This understanding reinforces commitment to the change process.

## 4. Start Small And Be Consistent

Initiate habit change by taking small, manageable steps. Starting small allows for gradual adaptation without overwhelming oneself. For instance, if the goal is to improve diet, begin by incorporating one extra serving of vegetables daily, gradually increasing the intake over time. Consistency in these small steps is key to building new habits.

## 5. Replace Harmful Habits With Positive Alternatives

Replace harmful habits with healthier alternatives. Identify and implement substitutes that align with your goals. For instance, replace sugary drinks with water or herbal teas, swap unhealthy snacks with fruits or nuts, or substitute sedentary activities with short walks or stretching exercises.

## 6. Use Behavioural Triggers And Cues And Stack Habits

Habit stacking is a simple way of using the habits we already have to help form new ones by attaching the new habit to an existing one. Stack habits by utilising existing habits as triggers or cues to prompt new habits. Create environmental cues that remind and motivate action. For instance, if the goal is to exercise in the morning, lay out workout clothes by the bed as a visual cue to initiate the activity upon waking. Another example is to say affirmations when you go to the bathroom to brush your teeth.

Affirmations are suggestions we can make about ourselves, to ourselves. For example if you wanted to be more confident you might start the day looking in the bathroom mirror saying "I am a confident and capable man". Over time the subconscious not only hears these suggestions but will start to integrate them, moving us towards the beliefs we want. This is part of the basis of hypnosis and NLP and affirmations are a powerful mental tool to have in your box. The key is to be consistent with them and to reinforce them – when you are feeling confident, remind yourself of that to reinforce the belief.

## 7. Create Accountability And Support Systems

Engage with a support system to enhance motivation and accountability.

Share goals and progress with a friend, family member, or support group. Accountability partners can offer encouragement, celebrate successes, and provide support during challenges.

## 8. Monitor Progress And Celebrate Success

Regularly track progress towards your set goals. Keep a journal, use apps, or employ other tracking methods to monitor changes. Celebrate small victories along the way—acknowledge and reward yourself for achieving milestones or making consistent efforts towards habit change.

## 9. Practise Self-Compassion And Patience

Embrace self-compassion and patience throughout the habit change process. Recognise that change takes time, and setbacks are part of the journey. Learn from setbacks without being too hard on yourself. Cultivate a positive mindset and focus on continual progress.

## 10. Seek Professional Guidance

Consider seeking guidance from professionals such as healthcare providers, nutritionists, or behavioural therapists. They can provide personalised strategies, practical advice, and support systems tailored to individual needs, facilitating successful habit change.

In conclusion, effectively changing habits requires a systematic approach that involves self-awareness, goal-setting, consistency, support systems, and patience.

By following these steps, individuals can gradually transition from harmful behaviours to positive habits, promoting better health, increased vitality, and optimised hormonal balance.

# PERFORMANCE PRINCIPLE 8: BUILDING A POSITIVE MINDSET

It's all about building a success mindset. Now you may already have that for business, for your career, even your relationships, but I see so many successful men who "fail" to believe they can be successful in their body goals. This is because our beliefs are so powerful and drive our behaviour, even subconsciously. There's a saying that if the acorn had the beliefs of a human, it would never become a nightly oak, and I love that. Our human mind is so powerful, but a lot of the software we run is inherited and just not appropriate for the goals we want to achieve.

The truth is that the one thing holding you back is you. You are defined by your self identity, none of us can outperform our self identity, which are our beliefs about who we are and what we can achieve. Like Henry Ford said, whether you think you can, or you think you can't, you're right.

That's a sobering thought. Without addressing our beliefs we're like the hamster running in the wheel, all action but never getting anywhere. You'll never truly thrive, if you don't change your beliefs about yourself. And this is where most people make the mistake...

You won't lose that belly fat. You won't feel confident in your skin. You won't feel powerful and capable, if you don't work on this crucial mindset shift. You'll stay stuck in that hamster wheel frustrated and disconnected.

## You Must Create A New Self Identity That's Aligned With Your Goals In Order To Achieve Long Term Success, Health And Happiness

I'm going to say that again because it's so important...

You must create a new self identity that's aligned with your goals in order to achieve long term success, health and happiness.

Most of our beliefs are not even ours, they were passed to us by our caregivers when we were children (usually our parents, but also teachers, etc.) or were shaped by events in our lives. Because they feel so intrinsically part of us we rarely question them, they are wrapped in our identity. But here's the thing, your beliefs are just a construct and while they might be "true" for you, they are just beliefs, not facts and you are allowed to not only question them, but question whether they are serving who you want to be.

We tend to think of our self identity or our beliefs as fixed things.

They're not, they're merely constructs and we can change them if we want to. In fact neuroscience shows us with the modern brain imaging technology, that our brain plasticity means our brain structure can actually change. So we can work to adopt new beliefs, and by doing that adopt a new self identity that's more aligned with who we want to be, than who we currently are.

Let me explain that a little more in simple terms. Our brain is both our hardware and our software. If we think of our thoughts, beliefs etc. as the software that's running, then we can think of the actual structure of the brain as our hardware. When we practise a habit or belief, we lay down a new neural pathway. The more we practise that thing the bigger the pathway, so our hardware is adapting to make our software more effective.

Well that's great when we have a helpful habit or belief, but when we have one we want to change, that's where we need to do the work. When we do our brain structure will change, remapping neural pathways for the new belief or habit.

This is why at times of stress for example, we may fall back into an old habit or belief, because the pathway is more ingrained. Even knowing this can allow us to have more compassion for ourselves, and knowing it means we can work on reinforcing the new habit or belief so that over time that becomes our default rather than the old one.

If the beliefs that we inherit are holding us back and they aren't even ours, why not choose new ones that are going to help you and support you to have the success that you want in life?

## A Basic Model Of Human Behaviour

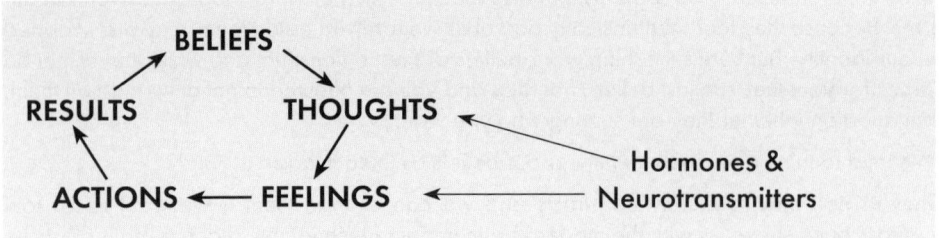

Here's a diagram of a basic model of human behaviour. We can jump in anywhere on the circle, so let's look at an example. Let's say I'm chased by a small dog as a child. As a result, I start to believe that all dogs are dangerous. So when I'm out as an adult, and I see a dog walking towards me, my thought is "Oh, no", I start to feel scared, I get nervous, the action is, I run away. The result is the dog starts chasing me and reinforces my belief that dogs are dangerous, even if it's a tiny little fluff ball that's just playing.

What that means for us in practice is we're always flicking between the present and the past. Because our subconscious doesn't have a linear concept of time, what's happening now is the same as what happened when you were a child years ago. Our brain is basically what I call an inference engine, we're exposed to so much stimulus, it cannot process it all. So it just attempts to fill in the gaps based on past experience. What our subconscious does is it flicks back to the past experience, when presented with a situation now, and bases our behaviour around that past event, so we spend our lives pinging between the past and the present. Which means if we haven't altered our neural software, we never get to our dream life.

The other thing I want to say on this is that we also need to be aware that because we've got these hormonal changes going on as well changes to levels of our testosterone primarily also our neurotransmitters, that's having an interference effect on our thoughts and feelings.

For example testosterone plays a role in confidence, so if levels are low we might have more anxiety. So this feedback loop is getting interfered with anyway. And that experience tends to be in a negative pattern. We're getting more anxious, maybe even more depressed. So knowing that we definitely want to take steps to reinforce ourselves with positive thoughts and start working towards this dream life.

Unfortunately one belief a lot of people have is that changing our beliefs is hard. Wrong. It's not easy, but change is possible. It takes work but changing our psychology delivers long term success and makes everything else so much easier. Once our beliefs and behaviours are aligned with our goal, and we take action, we become unstoppable.

One powerful way we can start to change our beliefs (and so our behaviours) is to start actively priming our subconscious for our new life by not just thinking about our future, but engaging in it by using tools from Neuro Linguistic Programming (NLP). A tool we use a lot we call future rehearsal. With future rehearsal instead of using our imaginations in the way we normally do, (for the worst outcomes!) we start actually using our imagination for the right purpose, to create where we want to be.

Again, neuroscience and modern scanning shows us that our brains can't distinguish between imagination if it's vivid enough, and reality so we can actually prep our brains for the future we want. I've got an example, if you've watched downhill skiers before they take the course, they'll be a top of the slope crouched down and actually swaying side to side mentally running the course first in their minds. In fact nearly all top performing sports people do this, they rehearse what they're going to do first in their minds and see themselves being successful.

We'll use a version of this writing a letter from our future self in the programme section.

We can also leverage a psychological theory which is another basic model of human behaviour called Congruence Theory. Congruence Theory states that our beliefs and our behaviours must be aligned for us to be in balance, when they're misaligned, we will experience a state of dissonance. Then when we're in dissonance with our beliefs and behaviours mismatched, either our belief or our behaviour will change to bring us back to a state of balance.

This theory is so powerful it underpins many types of overt and covert persuasion. If you identify with a particular belief then behaving contrary to it will cause you distress. For example, say you passionately believe in avoiding fast food but on a trip you have no option but to eat it as there's nothing else available, you're going to feel uncomfortable.

Likely you'll start to justify it to yourself, that there really was no other option, the food's not as bad as you thought. Or you'll make a commitment to never get caught out that way again, to plan snacks to take with you when you travel. In effect you'll adapt your beliefs to excuse your behaviour, or in future double down on your behaviour to support your beliefs. If you want to go to the dark side of it. This is also what they used when they started to experiment with brainwashing in the 60s and how they would do it was by getting people to take small steps with their belief and their behaviours. And then over time, they could change their whole belief structure. The great thing is we can use this for good to get the results we want for ourselves. We can use it to change our own beliefs and become the people that we want to be.

So how do we do that? Well our beliefs are stronger than our behaviour, our beliefs win most of the time, so we focus on changing the belief and reinforcing that with the new behaviour. This is why people fail on diets by the way. At some level they have a belief that they don't think they can sustain it, that it's not possible for them, and so the belief wins out, they give up and go back to their own ways. So changing your beliefs is crucial for change.

> *"Well our beliefs are stronger than our behaviour."*

Where many people go wrong is waiting for some ill-defined external event to impact how you feel about yourself and change your beliefs for you. You're going to be waiting a long time, your beliefs won't change on their own.

So what we need to do is leverage our psychology, we want to work on our beliefs and our behaviour at the same time to turbocharge your results. That means that you not only start to act like the person you want to become, but believe you're that person too. And that is how success is made and sustained. And this again, this is proven psychology. This is not faking it until you make it. This is committing to a new way of being and believing and constantly reinforcing it. It's about stepping into that future self identity.

I'm going to break it down in a different way for you. Most of us operate from a Have, Do, Be model. When I Have X, will Do Y, then I will Be Z.

For example, when I have more time, then I'll go to the gym more, then I'll have the body I want. Or when I have more time off from work, I'll work on that side hustle business plan and I'll make my millions.

The problem with this is twofold: firstly it means we're always delaying gratification to some point in the future — when I've got these other things in place, then I'll have this thing and then I'll allow myself to be happy.

Secondly we're not living as the person that already has that thing, so we're not working on our beliefs or behaviour. Instead we want to flip it around to Be, Do, Have.

I am a fit person because I'm going to the gym and I'm eating healthily. I am creating new wealth by working on my business plan by creating the time to do this.

When you switch it around like this you start living your new reality now. Your new beliefs and new behaviours are aligned and congruence theory means that they'll embed faster.

We can also accelerate our progress by spending time in our future via our imagination with tools like future rehearsal and by reinforcing with other tools like affirmations, but also by taking what we call energetic action. Energetic action is action not directly related towards your goals but aligned with them. You can imagine how someone who had your new beliefs and new self identity might act.

Do they take art classes because they want to explore that side of themselves? Do they volunteer? Do they read more books? You get the idea. These are all facets to building the new persona aligned with the ultimate goal.

Remember, you've "failed" in the past because you didn't know this stuff, and because you've waited for your beliefs to catch up with your reality, which is the single greatest mistake you can make, you'll be waiting a hell of a long time.

Now you have the power to shape your beliefs, your reality, your future.

One last word here and I would love you to take this away as a lesson for life: discipline is a super power. Discipline means doing the stuff you know you need to do but don't want to do, repeatedly.

If that sounds too hard, then think about the alternative... Sure it might seem difficult to devote some of your time to being fit and healthy, but how hard does it feel if you don't do the work and you end up fragile, ill and dying early?

Tip: When you're about to make a poor choice, pause and play it forward. What do you want your tomorrow to look like? Then choose.

Here's three secrets about discipline:

1. **You've probably already nailed discipline in one area of your life, likely something you enjoy. You'll do it pretty much no matter what. That means you've got the capability and you can map it into other areas of your life.**
2. **When you consciously apply discipline to an area of your life, you'll find that it starts to seep into other areas of your life too, meaning you will level up in multiple areas.**
3. **The more you practise discipline the easier it gets. Essentially you form a habit. Will there still be hard days? Absolutely but you'll find it easier than harder to do the right thing the majority of times.**

## CASE STUDY: **JOHN (48)**

When John first came to me, he was 48 and feeling stuck. His energy levels were at an all-time low, and it was affecting every aspect of his life. He had gained significant weight over the past few years and felt deeply unhappy with his body shape. This physical discomfort fed into his low self-esteem, leading him to withdraw socially and doubt his capabilities in both his personal and professional life. He described feeling "old before his time," lacking the motivation to take control of his health and unsure if change was even possible for him.

We began with a holistic approach, starting with small but impactful changes to his eating and exercise habits. First, I worked on a nutrition plan that focused on whole foods and balanced macronutrients, ensuring his body was fuelled properly to boost his energy levels and support weight loss. John had a history of fad dieting, so it was crucial to shift his mindset around food—from restriction and guilt to nourishment and sustainability.

I also introduced an exercise routine that was tailored to his lifestyle and fitness level. John hadn't been active in years, so we started with simple movements that were easy to stick to, gradually increasing intensity as his fitness improved. Over time, he began to enjoy working out, as he saw the positive effects on his body and energy levels.

But the most significant shift came in his mindset. Through NLP coaching techniques and daily practices, we worked on breaking down John's limiting beliefs, the ones that told him he wasn't capable of change or that it was too late for him. By reframing his thinking, I helped John see that he was in control of his own narrative. We set small, achievable goals to build his confidence and slowly, his self-perception began to shift. He started to believe in his ability to change, not just his body, but his entire approach to life.

Within a few weeks, John's body shape began to transform. He shed the excess weight, but more importantly, he started to feel stronger, more energised and healthier than he had in years. As his fitness improved, so did his confidence, he no longer felt like his body was holding him back.

John's newfound self-belief led to significant shifts in other areas of his life. He re-engaged socially, started being more go-getting at work and began pursuing hobbies he had previously abandoned due to lack of energy and motivation. His outlook on life had completely changed; he no longer saw midlife as a time of decline but as a new beginning, full of possibility. By changing his habits, both physically and mentally, John felt he had truly reclaimed his life.

His transformation wasn't just about weight loss—it was about rediscovering his potential, both inside and out.

# PERFORMANCE PRINCIPLE 9: CONNECTION, VALUES, PASSION AND PURPOSE

We're going to talk about creating emotional resilience, or if you'd rather, emotional wellbeing. So we often neglect what we could term spirituality, it's not woo-woo though, again, the benefits are rooted in neuroscience and research.

At its roots, it's really important to say that spirituality is NOT religion. Some people are religious, if religion is your thing, then that's great. But spirituality doesn't mean religion. Rather it's a sense of connection to the self to others or to a higher power.

We have three basic spiritual needs:

- to be seen
- to be heard
- to matter

When we feel that these needs are met, when we have a connection to ourselves or to a deeper purpose, then we can gain a healthier set of perspectives on our purpose in life.

And this is something to consider – what are your values? What is your legacy? What do you want to leave behind?

What is the story of your life that you wish to tell? And most importantly, what is the cost of your inaction and not taking steps towards that?

It's human nature to ignore or discount the cost of staying stuck where you are (the opportunity cost) and instead focus on the cost of the action we're thinking of taking, and evaluating whether it has a pay off or not. So for example, you're overweight and that makes you miserable and is impacting your health, but when you think about adjusting your nutrition and moving your body more to lose the weight, you focus on the discipline you'll need, the foods you love you'll miss out

> *"What is the story of your life that you wish to tell? And most importantly, what is the cost of your inaction and not taking steps towards that?"*

on, how hard it will be and talk yourself out of it, rather than focusing on how your life will be improved when you get the result.

Because we often neglect that opportunity cost of not doing the thing, we tend to always think about what this might cost me if it goes wrong, what it will cost us if we fail. Then compounding that we also discount the pain and discomfort in right now staying where we are.

Here's one tip I can share with you. And again, there's a lot of work on this in the fields of positive psychology about working with gratitude. As the wonderful Neale Donald Walsh says, "The struggle ends when gratitude begins."

According to research from the Universities of California and of Miami, grateful people are less likely to feel sick or get sick or feel depressed. And they're more likely to exercise. In relationships showing gratitude promotes more positive feelings, and helps people feel more comfortable expressing their emotions to each other.

An attitude of gratitude is shown to raise serotonin and dopamine, the feel good neurotransmitters that help promote better sleep, greater mental resilience and reduce your stress levels. So one of the most simple things you can do that will make a difference to how you feel emotionally is to start working with gratitude. And this is about focusing on what you're grateful for in your life.

You can't be in gratitude and fear or resentment at the same time, they're opposing states, which is why a gratitude practice is so powerful and a great way to start your day.

So many of us are caught up with, "I'll be happy when…" No. Be happy now, don't make happiness a destination in the future. If you can't learn to be happy now, guess what, you won't be happy in the future either because you'll still be with the 'you of right now'.

Be honest, how many times have you thought that? "When I buy that new thing, won't that be amazing. I'll be happy."

It could be a car, a watch, an outfit, a holiday. There's that momentary happiness then you're like, "Oh, what's the next thing?"

To slow this constant need for more, you should start practising gratitude. A really simple way to do that is a morning ritual.

It takes less than 5 minutes. First thing, before you let the world in, before you look at your phone, turn on the TV, before you start the day, take some time for you. Grab a pen and paper and simply write down three things you're grateful for from the day before. Three things you're grateful for generally in your life, and an intention for the day, I get all our clients to do this. They all report massive shifts in their positivity over time. It really really does work.

Related to gratitude and to stress is remembering that you have the power to choose your reaction when someone or something is pushing your buttons. If you have a trigger that you know you could either remove (remove it) or if you can't remove, that you could choose a different reaction to so that you're not negatively impacted, then choose the different reaction! A great example here is social media. If someone is always posting stuff that annoys you, unfriend them or snooze them – trigger removed. You haven't lost, you've won, you have peace of mind.

You know, doing the same thing over and over again, is the definition of insanity. So do something different, you may surprise you, and the other person! It sounds challenging, I get it, you end up getting in that same stress situation, it keeps occurring with this person, (maybe it's the dishes, the laundry, whatever) and you can't remove that person from your life because that's not always practical. So choose a different reaction. Choose harmony for you.

It's hard, easier said than done. But we can train ourselves to do that. And when you do these things and you start to incorporate them you'll begin to notice a huge shift in your energy. Here's a little tip, if you feel a situation spiralling and you don't like how you're feeling ask yourself this question:

Do you want to be right or do you want to be happy?

The answer will be your guide as to what to do...

Now let's delve deeper into the significance of connection, values, passion, and purpose at midlife:

## 1. Connection And Social Relationships

Cultivating Meaningful Relationships:

At midlife, maintaining strong social connections becomes crucial. Cultivating meaningful relationships with friends, family, or community groups fosters a sense of belonging and emotional support. These connections provide companionship, empathy, and a support network during life's ups and downs. Having a strong network means we feel supported, we have a place to voice ideas, get feedback, build accountability and connect with like-minded others. As well as feeling like we belong good networks can also bring opportunities, resources, direction and meaning. All too often men can end up isolated in later life through failing to build and maintain their networks – note guys – this means out of work too! When you retire you want a network around you, you don't want to be starting from scratch. So, do network for your career or business, but network around hobbies, sports, interests so that you have a varied and durable selection of friends and contacts.

### Impact on Mental and Emotional Health:
Strong social bonds positively impact mental and emotional health. Studies show that individuals with robust social networks often experience reduced stress, increased happiness, and a lower risk of mental health issues. Sharing experiences and emotions with others offers comfort and resilience during challenging times.

## 2. Values Clarification

### Reflecting on Personal Beliefs:
Midlife prompts introspection about personal beliefs and principles. Now you may be one of the lucky ones who knows what your core values are, and abides by them, but many of us aren't really aware of what they are. One exercise you can do is make a list of 10 values you feel are important to you, listing out things such as freedom, justice, equality, wealth... Once you have your 10, discard half of them (not as easy as it sounds). Then whittle down to a final three. These are your core values. Reflect whether these are what you're currently living, or if you need to make some changes to embody them more in your life. Clarifying core values helps in making decisions aligned with one's authentic self. This introspection guides life choices, promotes a sense of integrity, and fosters authenticity in actions and interactions.

### Guiding Life Choices:
When decisions and actions align with one's values, it leads to a greater sense of satisfaction and fulfilment. Living in harmony with one's values promotes a sense of purpose and direction, contributing to a more meaningful life.

## 3. Rediscovering Passion

### Exploring Interests and Hobbies:
Midlife offers an opportunity to explore or reignite passions and interests. Engaging in hobbies, creative pursuits, or activities that bring joy fosters personal growth and mental stimulation. Pursuing passions provides a sense of fulfilment, creativity, and adds vibrancy to daily life.

### Source of Personal Fulfilment:
Embracing passions contributes to a sense of personal fulfilment and satisfaction. It allows individuals to dedicate time to activities that bring them joy, helping them maintain a healthy work-life balance and overall wellbeing.

## 4. Defining Purpose

Finding Meaning and Direction:

Having a sense of purpose gives meaning and direction to life. It involves setting meaningful goals, contributing to society, or pursuing ambitions that align with personal values and passions. Defining purpose provides a compass for navigating life's challenges and transitions.

Motivation and Resilience:

A clear sense of purpose fuels motivation and resilience during challenging times. It instills a sense of drive and determination, enabling individuals to overcome obstacles and setbacks with optimism and perseverance.

## 5. Maintaining Emotional Wellbeing

Intersection of Connection, Values, Passion, and Purpose:

The interplay between connection, aligned values, pursued passions, and a sense of purpose contributes to emotional wellbeing. Building relationships, living authentically, engaging in meaningful activities, and having a clear direction in life promote mental health and life satisfaction.

Holistic Impact on Wellbeing:

The holistic impact of these elements leads to reduced stress, improved mental health, increased life satisfaction, and a greater sense of fulfilment. This holistic approach supports overall wellbeing across various aspects of life.

At midlife, nurturing connections, clarifying values, embracing passions, and defining purpose collectively contribute to a rich and fulfilling life. Integrating these elements creates a framework for resilience, personal growth, and a more meaningful life experience.

I can't stress enough how much creating a passion or purpose for your life, aligning your values with it and choosing a different reaction to keep you in gratitude, and how daily practice of gratitude will positively impact your life. Get to it.

This is something you have to work at though, you can't do an exercise once or twice and expect a difference. However, daily practice with the exercises, then what I call "active practice" can really move the needle fast. Active practice is when you become aware of acknowledging moments of gratitude, when you're aligned with your values, your emotions etc. as you go through the day, rather than just sailing through your day somewhat unaware. This helps us to live in a way more aligned with who we want to be, rather than who we are currently and over time we step more and more into that future version of ourselves as we embody the behaviours, beliefs, values and emotions of that person.

When we do this we're actually rewiring our neural pathways to create the new thought patterns so over time it becomes our natural behaviour.

Practise it, you'll be pleasantly surprised.

# PERFORMANCE PRINCIPLE 10: SUPPLEMENTS

I'd love to tell you that there's a natural, inexpensive herbal supplement you could take that would instantly boost your testosterone and give you more energy, a raging libido, and all the things you've probably seen advertised on social media... But, I'm all about honesty, and sadly, that supplement does NOT exist. So don't waste your money on things you see online with big promises, you'll only end up poorer and disappointed.

Having said that, there are some supplements that will support good hormone health, overall good health, and help reduce cortisol and possibly slightly boost testosterone.

It goes without saying that you want to ensure you're getting enough of the right vitamins and minerals to support good hormone and in particular, testosterone health: vitamins C and D both play a role in hormone support as do the minerals zinc and magnesium, so ensure you're getting enough of these and consider supplementation. Adaptogens such as Ashwagandha can also help balance hormone levels, including levels of the stress hormone cortisol. Adaptogens are simply natural substances (herbs) considered to help the body adapt to stress.

Here's a run down of supplements that can help when combined with a healthy diet and lifestyle:

## 1. Ashwagandha

Cortisol Suppression: Ashwagandha, an adaptogenic herb, has shown promising results in reducing cortisol levels. Studies suggest that it helps manage stress by modulating the body's stress response, thereby lowering cortisol production.

Testosterone Support: Research indicates that Ashwagandha may also support healthy testosterone levels. It seems to positively impact testosterone production and reproductive health in men.

## 2. Rhodiola Rosea

Cortisol Suppression: Rhodiola Rosea is another adaptogenic herb known for its stress-reducing properties. Studies suggest it may help lower cortisol levels, thereby mitigating the negative effects of stress on the body.

Testosterone Support: While more research is needed, some studies suggest that Rhodiola Rosea may contribute to improving testosterone levels by reducing stress-related hormone imbalances.

## 3. Magnesium

Cortisol Suppression: Magnesium plays a role in stress regulation and may help in reducing cortisol levels. Adequate magnesium intake has been associated with lower stress responses and improved mood.

Testosterone Support: Studies have indicated that magnesium supplementation might support healthy testosterone levels, particularly in individuals with deficiencies.

## 4. Vitamin D

Cortisol Suppression: Vitamin D deficiency has been linked to higher cortisol levels. Adequate vitamin D levels are associated with better stress regulation and reduced cortisol production.

Testosterone Support: Vitamin D supplementation has shown potential in supporting healthy testosterone levels, especially in individuals with vitamin D deficiencies.

Two other herbs that some swear by, but where the research is mixed are Tongkat Ali (sometimes called Long Jack) and Maca. Tongkat Ali has long been touted as a testosterone booster, but in fact studies have shown that it may be the suppressive effect on cortisol that allows great testosterone production.

Maca hasn't been shown to increase testosterone levels but seems to promote a healthy hormone balance, and users frequently report increased energy levels.

Try them and see how you get on as we all have individual responses to different supplements.

# BONUS PRINCIPLE: ACCOUNTABILITY

Maybe you can do this on your own. Maybe. Why not massively increase your chances of success? Here's an unpopular truth, motivation is finite.

Research shows us we have a pool of motivation, which gradually drains through the day as we use it up. So, of course there are times we're going to find it hard, times that it becomes too tough to keep going, even if we really want to achieve a goal.

Even if you have knowledge in the area you are working on and the tools you need to succeed, nothing beats having someone to cheer you on, show you the way and keep you on track.

Accountability is so, so important. Despite being a coach myself, I'm always working with at least one coach to help me stay focussed on areas I want to experience growth or change in. In fact, right now, I'm working with four coaches across different areas of my life. Why? Because going out alone is tough.

A while back I fooled myself that I could do it without support, so I took a break from having a coach for five months. Guess what? I noticed so much in my world started to slide. Even though I was set up, I had the tools and the strategy, I couldn't stay fully motivated as I was lacking that external accountability. As soon as I committed to a coach again, everything picked up. Everything.

Think back to a time when you set out to achieve something, but failed as you lost motivation or found it too hard going out alone?

Here's the painful truth, if you're not where you want to be, if you haven't managed to change it on your own by now, then the chances are you're not going to make it unless you feel supported and encouraged to do so.

Sorry to be blunt but that's how it is. And it is also completely natural.

That is why, I always recommend a mentor. It can be a friend or a trainer, or if that is not accessible for you, I will be your mentor from the pages of this book. It can be enough to have the knowledge that you are not the only one following this path, that you are not the only one needing to change, to encourage you to complete the course.

You've taken a massive first step, as you're holding this book in your hands. It's giving you not just a ton of knowledge and practical tools and actions, but a proven blueprint.

The fact is, when we commit to someone else, we're much more likely to succeed at our goal. We need someone in our corner that's been there and done it, that can guide others to the goal, that has life experience.

Someone who's going to talk through fears and struggles, who's going to celebrate the wins with you, who's going to keep you accountable and be the lighthouse that illuminates your path to success.

A good mentor will educate you and inspire you. They've got the tools, they're going to give you the confidence by allowing you to borrow their belief, just as I am now. After all, I have done this before, many times and I am confident it will work for you, as it has for others, providing you stay the course.

If you don't have the belief right now that you can make it, borrow mine. I am happy to lend it. I believe in you and you believe in me, so let's spread that belief around. There is real power in that.

*"If you don't have the belief right now that you can make it, borrow mine. I am happy to lend it. I believe in you and you believe in me, so let's spread that belief around. There is real power in that."*

If you want to take it one step further, you can do things like get accountability buddies, you can join communities, either virtually or in real life and they are useful tools. Even better, if it is possible, I would always suggest investing in coaching or mentoring. From my own personal experience, when you actually have skin in the game, that's when you become super accountable and the motivation rolls in.

# A Summary Of The Principles

*That's the theory, and the action steps for you to take. And I emphasise that, for you to take. Remember, nothing changes if nothing changes. If you read this book and don't take action, then you're not staying as you are, these andropause processes are happening anyway, so you'll actually be going backwards, and no one wants that.*

Maybe you think it sounds too hard? I'll tell you what's hard: watching your strength and energy go. Watching yourself shift to a negative mindset. Watching your ambition and motivation go. Watching your relationships fall apart.

I'm being bleak, but if you don't do something about this NOW it is bleak.

The good news is that you don't have to do a whole lot. This isn't about making massive wholesale changes in your life, it's about making small multiple changes that add up over time to make a BIG difference.

You don't need to live like a monk, exercise to exhaustion, eat salad for every meal. What you need to do is follow the advice given, follow the 30-day programme and incorporate these small changes into your life. Small sacrifices, big positive results.

Do not leave it until it's too late, the sooner you can make a start on this the better. I've worked with clients in their mid-60s who were exhausted, out of shape, out of love with life, and they have turned it around to launch new businesses, reignite their relationship, go out and do amazing things while feeling more energised than they did in their 20s, so it's possible, but only if you commit.

So, do you want a life that's lost its sparkle, where you've lost your shine? Or do you want to embrace your potential and do what it takes to get there?

There you have 10 Performance Principles (and your bonus principle Accountability), principles you can adapt into your life which will make a positive difference to your energy levels, how you feel, your physique and your mental state.

Each of these is designed to allow you to make small tweaks to your lifestyle rather than wholesale disruptive changes. The more you can adapt the better, but remember, something is better than nothing, so start with what feels achievable for you. Be kind to yourself and remember, you've got this!

## But...

Some of you will have read this far and thought, "Hell yeah! I want to get going!"

That's great, but I also know that some of you will already be thinking along the lines of, "Well it sounds great, but I don't know if I have the time, or the energy right now... what if it doesn't work for me...?" And so on.

Listen, it's natural to have objections, as humans we're wired to fear change, but how's your life right now? How does it look down the line in 6 months, a year, two years if you do nothing?

The truth is, what I've laid out won't take huge chunks of time out your life and it won't cost you much, but it will make a difference to your quality of life. So why not at least try it, or even better commit to it?

I'm going to break down those objections for you now...

# Objection
## "I Don't Have Time."

*Be honest, this is perhaps the weakest excuse. We can find the time if it matters. How long are you spending watching TV? Looking at your phone?*

I get it, the daily grind, the demands of work, and the ever-pressing obligations to family and commitments can create a narrative that self-care is a luxury we can ill afford. But here's the emotional truth: if we don't make time, nothing changes.

The reality is that the ticking clock is indifferent to our wellbeing. It continues its steady cadence, often drowning out the whispers of our internal health needs. In the midst of this hustle, the choice to prioritise our health becomes not just a practical decision but an emotional one. It's a declaration that our wellbeing matters, that our vitality deserves a seat at the table of priorities.

### Micro-Adjustments For Macro Impact:
Understanding that significant changes can stem from small, consistent actions is pivotal. Instead of envisioning a complete overhaul of your schedule, consider incorporating micro-adjustments as laid out in this book, for example, this could be as simple as taking a few minutes each morning for deep breathing exercises or choosing nutrient-dense snacks over processed ones.

### Efficiency In Exercise:
Transforming your body doesn't necessarily demand hours in the gym. High-intensity interval training (HIIT) and short, focused workouts can be incredibly effective. These can be completed in a fraction of the time but deliver impactful results. It's about quality over quantity.

## Strategic Time Management:
Taking a closer look at your daily schedule is a key step. Identify pockets of time that can be optimised. It might be during your lunch break, early morning, or even in the evening. Designate specific times for self-care, whether it's preparing a nutritious meal, engaging in a brief workout, or practicing mindfulness.

## Incorporate Wellness Into Daily Tasks:
Multitasking can work in your favour when it comes to wellbeing. Use moments of waiting or routine activities to your advantage. Listen to informative podcasts or audiobooks about andropause while commuting, or practise stress-relief techniques during short breaks at work.

## Set Realistic Expectations:
Acknowledge that transformation is a gradual process. Setting unrealistic expectations can lead to feelings of overwhelm. Instead, focus on achievable goals within the constraints of your current schedule. As you experience positive changes, you may find more motivation to carve out additional time.

## Prioritise Self-Care As A Non-Negotiable:
Shift the mindset around self-care from being optional to a non-negotiable aspect of your routine. When we recognise the importance of our wellbeing, we naturally make room for it in our schedules. Remember, investing time in yourself is an investment in a healthier, more fulfilling future.

## Build Consistency Over Intensity:
Consistency trumps intensity. Rather than occasional marathon efforts, aim for a regular, sustainable routine. Even short, daily rituals focused on wellbeing can accumulate into profound transformations over time. Discipline really is a super power.

In the grand tapestry of life, the threads of self-care should weave seamlessly into the narrative. If we don't make time, if we don't prioritise our wellbeing, the story remains unchanged. But if we dare to carve out those intentional moments, we unfurl a new chapter – a chapter where health, vitality, and a fulfilling life take centre stage.

# Objection
## "I Can't Afford To Do It."

*You can spend as much or as little as you want. The misconception that self-care comes with a hefty price tag often becomes a stumbling block.*

However, the pursuit of wellbeing need not be synonymous with financial strain. Here's how we can navigate the path to transformation even when financial resources are limited.

### Mindful Investment In Health:
Investing in your wellbeing doesn't always translate to exorbitant expenses. Rather than viewing it as a financial burden, consider it a mindful investment in your long-term health. By prioritising wellness now, you may prevent potential health issues that could lead to more significant financial burdens down the road.

### Accessible Nutrition:
Nutrient-dense foods need not break the bank. Embrace cost-effective staples such as whole grains, legumes, and seasonal fruits and vegetables. Strategic meal planning and opting for home-cooked meals can be both economical and beneficial for your overall health.

### Budget-Friendly Exercise Options:
Physical activity doesn't require an expensive gym membership. Explore budget-friendly options such as walking, jogging, or engaging in bodyweight exercises at home like I've laid out in Part 2. The key is to find activities that align with your budget while promoting an active lifestyle.

## Prioritise Essentials:

When resources are limited, focus on the essentials. Prioritise activities and interventions that have the most significant impact on your wellbeing. This might include investing in foundational aspects such as nutritious food, regular physical activity, and stress-management techniques.

## Community Support And Shared Resources:

Communities often offer shared resources and support. Look for local groups, online forums, or community events that focus on wellness. Shared experiences and knowledge can be invaluable, providing a sense of community without the need for significant financial investment.

## Explore Affordable Supplements:

Supplements that support andropause management need not be extravagant. Affordable options such as vitamin D, magnesium, and omega-3 fatty acids can be beneficial. Consult with healthcare professionals to identify cost-effective yet impactful supplement choices.

## Financial Planning For Wellness:

Consider incorporating wellness into your financial planning. Allocate a specific budget for health-related expenses, and explore cost-effective alternatives for achieving your wellness goals. This proactive approach aligns your financial priorities with your commitment to wellbeing.

## Negotiating Affordable Healthcare:

If you're going down the private route (in the UK we have free healthcare), explore options for affordable healthcare. Look into community health clinics, public health programmes, or insurance plans that cater to your budget. Negotiate costs where possible and communicate openly with healthcare providers about your financial constraints.

Don't make false savings – what's it going to cost you down the line NOT to take action?

# Objection
## "I Just Don't Have The Energy To Do This."

*Yep, I get it. The fatigue that comes with hormonal changes can cast a shadow on the prospect of embarking on a transformative journey.*

However, it's important to recognise that reclaiming vitality doesn't require an overwhelming burst of energy. It can be about small steps over time that lead to significant changes. I've helped men with chronic fatigue syndrome transform their bodies, their energy levels, getting them out running distances they never thought they'd do. So it is possible for you too.

### Micro-Changes For Macro Energy:
Acknowledge that significant transformations often arise from small, consistent changes. Rather than aiming for monumental shifts, focus on micro-adjustments that align with your current energy levels. This could be as simple as incorporating short walks into your routine or choosing energy-boosting snacks.

### Gentle Exercise To Recharge:
Exercise doesn't have to be exhaustive to be effective. I've laid out short but effective exercise protocols for you in the second part of the book. You do not need to be spending hours a day exercising to get great results and in fact in midlife and beyond, in fact more is often counter-productive as you'll elicit a stress response which works against what you're trying to achieve.

## Strategic Time Management:

Optimise your daily schedule to align with your energy peaks. Identify times when your energy is naturally higher, and reserve those moments for activities that require more focus or physical exertion. By strategically managing your time, you can make the most of your available energy reservoir.

## Nutrient-Dense Fuel:

Consider your diet as a source of energy. Nutrient-dense foods, including whole grains, lean proteins, and a variety of colourful fruits and vegetables, can provide sustained energy throughout the day. Hydration is also crucial, as even mild dehydration can contribute to feelings of fatigue.

## Prioritise Rest And Recovery:

Acknowledge the importance of rest in the overall energy equation. Quality sleep and moments of intentional relaxation are essential for hormonal balance and energy restoration. Prioritise a consistent sleep schedule and create a bedtime routine that promotes restful sleep.

## Mindful Stress Management:

Chronic stress can drain your energy reservoir. Incorporate mindful stress management techniques such as deep breathing, meditation, or engaging in activities that bring joy. Managing stress not only conserves energy but also contributes to a more balanced hormonal profile.

## Social Support For Energy Boost:

Surround yourself with a supportive community. Positive social interactions can be energising and uplifting. Share your goals with friends, family or a support group, and draw on the collective energy of those cheering you on.

## Set Realistic Expectations:

Recognise that the path to wellbeing is a journey, not a sprint. Setting realistic expectations for yourself is crucial, preventing feelings of overwhelm and fatigue. Celebrate small victories along the way, acknowledging the energy and effort you invest in your wellbeing.

## Professional Guidance For Personalised Energy Solutions:

Consider seeking guidance from healthcare professionals or wellness experts (like me). They can help tailor strategies to your unique energy profile, addressing potential underlying factors contributing to fatigue and providing personalised solutions.

Reclaiming energy is not about a sudden surge but a gradual, intentional process. By approaching your wellbeing with compassion, strategic choices, and small manageable steps, you can lay the foundation for renewed vitality. Remember, each step forward is a testament to your commitment to a life infused with energy and wellbeing.

# Objection
## "I Don't Believe In Myself To Make Changes Or To See This Through."

*You can borrow belief, borrow it from this book, borrow it from me, borrow it from people you see around you that are making changes. Borrow that belief until you start getting the results that build your own belief, because it will come. Self-belief is a skill that can be nurtured and strengthened. Let's explore how you can cultivate that self-belief.*

### Acknowledge The Power Of Self-Compassion:
Begin by acknowledging that change is a process, and setbacks are a natural part of any journey. Replace self-criticism with self-compassion. Understand that life is not about perfection but about progress and self-care.

## Break Down Goals Into Manageable Steps:

Rather than viewing the entire journey as a mountain to climb, break it down into smaller, more manageable steps. By setting achievable goals, you can create a series of victories that build confidence over time. For example, if you were going to set out to build a house from scratch, you wouldn't just get bricks and start building. You'd draft plans, work out the plumbing, the wiring, step by step you'd create the new home. If we're going for a goal we've never achieved before it can seem overwhelming, so break it down into micro goals and focus on the next step.

## Draw Inspiration From Past Achievements:

Reflect on past achievements, no matter how small they may seem. Whether it's overcoming a challenge at work or successfully navigating a personal obstacle, these experiences highlight your resilience and capability. Use them as a source of inspiration for the changes ahead.

## Create A Supportive Environment:

Surround yourself with individuals who believe in your potential. Share your goals with friends, family, or a support group. Positive affirmations and encouragement from those around you can reinforce your belief in your capacity for change.

## Visualise For Success:

Practise visualisation techniques where you vividly imagine yourself succeeding in your goals. Envision the positive impact of the changes you're making and how it enhances your overall wellbeing. Really connect with the emotion of you succeeding at your goals.

## Mindful Affirmations:

Incorporate positive affirmations into your daily routine. Affirmations that reinforce your capability, resilience, and commitment to change can gradually shift your internal dialogue. Repeat these affirmations regularly to cultivate a more positive and self-affirming mindset.

## Learn From Setbacks As Opportunities:

I call this the shift from obstacle to opportunity thinking. Instead of viewing setbacks as failures, perceive them as opportunities for learning and growth. Understand that challenges are a natural part of any transformative journey. Analyse setbacks with a compassionate lens, extracting lessons that can guide you forward.

## Seek Professional Guidance:

Consider seeking guidance from professionals who specialise in andropause management, such as healthcare providers or wellness experts. Their expertise can provide you with tailored strategies, and their support can be instrumental in building belief in your ability to make positive changes.

## Connect With Others On Similar Journeys:

Joining a community of individuals facing similar challenges can foster a sense of shared experience. Engaging with others who are navigating andropause can provide mutual support, shared insights, and a reminder that you're not alone in your journey.

## Celebrate Your Progress:

Celebrate every milestone, no matter how small. Each step forward, each positive change, is a reason to celebrate. Acknowledging your progress reinforces the belief that you are capable of making meaningful changes in your life.

Remember, belief in oneself isn't a fixed trait but a dynamic skill that can be cultivated and strengthened over time. By embracing a mindset of self-compassion, breaking down goals, seeking support, and celebrating victories, you can gradually nurture the belief that will carry you through the transformative journey of andropause.

# Objection
## "I Don't Believe In The Process Enough."

*Doubting the effectiveness of the process is a common hurdle, but understanding and believing in the steps you're taking is integral to success.*

You've already taken the first steps by reading this book, you understand more than you did, awareness precedes change, so become more aware and look at the results others are getting – you're not that different.

### Educate Yourself:
Knowledge is a powerful antidote to scepticism. Dive deep into understanding the science behind andropause, the hormonal changes, and the proven strategies for managing its effects. The more you educate yourself, the more tangible and real the process becomes.

### Consult With Experts:
Engage with healthcare professionals, wellness experts, or specialists in andropause management. Their expertise provides valuable insights into the process, and they can offer personalised guidance based on your unique circumstances. A professional perspective can instil confidence in the effectiveness of the strategies.

### Set Realistic Expectations:
Clarify and set realistic expectations for the process. Understand that transformations take time, and results may not be immediate. By having realistic expectations, you create a foundation for patience and perseverance, essential elements of any successful journey.

## Track Your Progress:

Implement a system to track and monitor your progress. This could involve keeping a journal, using a health app or having regular check-ins with a healthcare professional. Tangible evidence of your advancements reinforces your belief in the process.

## Celebrate Wins:

Acknowledge and celebrate wins when you get results. Even small victories contribute to the overall success of the journey. By recognising and celebrating progress, you build confidence in the incremental effectiveness of the process.

## Join Supportive Communities:

Connect with communities or support groups focused on andropause or similar health journeys. Engaging with others who are following a similar process can provide shared insights, encouragement and a sense of collective belief in what you're doing, and who can help you celebrate your wins.

## Visualise The Future You:

Envision the future version of yourself who has already succeeded and got the results. Visualisation can be a powerful tool for building confidence. Picture the positive changes, the vitality, and the sense of wellbeing that the process is designed to bring.

## Adapt And Evolve:

Understand that the process is not static. It may require adaptation based on your individual responses and needs. The flexibility to adjust the approach fosters belief, as it reflects a process that is responsive and tailored to your unique journey.

By immersing yourself in knowledge, drawing inspiration from success stories, consulting with experts, and engaging with the process through experimentation, you can gradually build confidence in its effectiveness. Remember, belief in the process is not only about the steps you're taking but also about the belief you cultivate in your ability to achieve a healthier and more fulfilling life through andropause transformation.

Now, I can't force you to make the lifestyle changes laid out in this book but why would you not?

# Ask Yourself This

*So ask yourself this. You want to make a change. If you're sure that your risk would work out, how would you feel and behave?*

We often use our imagination for the worst outcomes. We imagine everything going wrong, we fear we might look foolish which is our ego talking. We don't stop to think about what it will be like if it works. We don't think, "How amazing would it be if it works? Oh my god, what would my life be like if it actually succeeded at that?"

The other thing we fail to do is to look at the opportunity cost. What's it costing me staying stuck here right now in this place?

And so in one year's time, what's the cost of my happiness, my bank account, my relationship, my children's lives, my health, if I don't take a step.

So here's my challenge to you. What small thing can you do in the next 48 hours to boost your confidence and take you towards a step that will make you take an even bigger risk and fundamentally change your life.

What can you do in the next 48 hours? Commit to it, and do it. You have nothing to lose and plenty to gain.

# ACTIONABLE STEPS TO START MAKING A DIFFERENCE NOW

So what are the next things you can do? Well in the second part of this book you have a complete 30-day programme, but I also want to leave you with actionable tips, here are my recommendations:

## Look At Your Life Equilibrium Right Now.
- Where are you expending your energy?
- Where do you need to focus more energy?

## We Always Think We've Got Tomorrow, We May Not Have.
So it's really important. We get straight on to where we want to spend our energy. Where's the gap now and how are you going to close it?

## Give Yourself A Realistic Outcome.
Think about your lifestyle, the goal you want, what you're willing to sacrifice and getting the balance so you are happy now.

## Make A Plan To Achieve It And Execute On It.

## Be Aware Of Your Midlife Hormones And Learn To Work With Them.

## You Must, Must, Must Get Your Stress And Your Cortisol Under Control.
I can't emphasise that strongly enough.
- So, learn stress management techniques
- Practise them, put them into action
- Learn your triggers
- Pick different reactions

## Start Moving Your Body Regularly

You must resistance train and give yourself adequate recovery. In The Midlife Reset we deliver a whole midlife specific workout programme that's progressive and has gym or home options. So it's tailored to your lifestyle and just fits around everything you're doing. The programme in the next section will also do the job though.

## Transition To A Healthy Diet

- High in whole foods
- Protein
- Healthy fats
- Natural carbs

In the next section this is all laid out for you, you can use the nutritional coaching tools I provide to really free yourself up around food for the long term.

That's how you'll make changes and sustain them. We have clients literally say after four weeks, "My relationship with food has completely transformed. I know what I should be eating and I know what I could be eating. I don't worry about that big blowout meal now as I know what to do around it."

Get those nutrition basics bedded in to understand what a good healthy diet should look like.

Work on your mindset to build a positive outlook, being present, having more fun in your life. Otherwise, life's just passing you by. This is about building that bulletproof mindset for success.

Start building your emotional resilience, I've outlined some tools, there are more daily tools in the programme section.

Get accountable. If you're not going to get a coach or mentor to work with, I strongly recommend that you do at least get a buddy or getting a group to help you take action. So many times we say to ourselves, "I'll do it tomorrow. I'll do it after my holiday. I'll do it after that party."

Start taking action now. Just think if you'd started this journey two weeks ago, where would you be now? Can you afford to keep putting it off, remind yourself of the cost of inaction and move forward, I can tell you once you do start moving momentum breeds momentum.

Taking these initial steps is an act of profound courage. It's a declaration to yourself that you are worthy of a life enriched with vitality, joy and purpose. The courage to embrace change, to confront the unknown is the catalyst that propels you toward the transformative horizon.

As you stand on the verge of this transformative journey, know that what lies ahead is not just a series of changes but a promise – a promise of a richer, more vibrant life and a version of yourself that is stronger, wiser, and more alive.

So, let's get going and let's take those first steps to your transformation and a more positive and fulfilling life.

# Part 2
## The 30-day Programme

# The 30-day Programme Introduction

*Welcome to the second part of the book which is a 30-day programme designed to get the foundations we've already looked at locked in. The programme has four components: nutrition, exercise, mindset and accountability.*

Now, this is going to help you with andropause, but it's all also going to help you in multiple areas of your life. We're interconnected beings, and just doing workouts or going on a diet isn't enough. We need something that's going to change our inner world too. That's what this is.

We know that hormonal and neurotransmitter changes are affecting our psychology, we know that our life experience has shaped our beliefs, and if those changes to our psychology aren't supporting us, then it's time to change them.

If you're unsure about this aspect then I ask you only to suspend your disbelief for 30-days, follow the programme and see what happens...

You will be pleasantly surprised.

Remember, do not pick and choose what you want to do, follow the whole thing. It won't take up much time and energy, it's just 30-days, and the results will be worth it.

I suggest you read through the entire programme and then start applying the nutrition learnings straight away. You have a four week exercise programme, and a four week mindset programme. DO NOT neglect any part of this. As we've already seen, we're holistic beings and this needs to work across every level.

It's designed to be easy to follow, time efficient and by making multiple small changes rather than large ones, it won't overwhelm you, but it will get results.

To access free resources accompanying this book, including links to podcasts, videos, workouts and nutrition information, head to themidlifementors.com/manual or scan this QR Code.

# Plan Summary

## Your 30-day Programme

**WEEK 1**

| AREA | DAY 1 | DAY 2 | DAY 3 |
|---|---|---|---|
| **Daily Practice** | Set your goals and make sure you're ready to go with everything you need | Daily Gratitude | Daily Gratitude |
| **Workouts** | Rest | Resistance Session 1 | HIIT Session |
| **Mindset** | Work on your Life Equlibirium | | |

**WEEK 2**

| AREA | DAY 8 | DAY 9 | DAY 10 |
|---|---|---|---|
| **Daily Practice** | Daily Gratitude | Daily Gratitude | Daily Gratitude |
| **Workouts** | Rest | Resistance Session 1 | HIIT Session |
| **Mindset** | Review Progress Towards Your Goals | | |

**WEEK 3**

| AREA | DAY 15 | DAY 16 | DAY 17 |
|---|---|---|---|
| **Daily Practice** | Daily Gratitude | Daily Gratitude | Daily Gratitude |
| **Workouts** | Rest | Resistance Session 1 | HIIT Session |
| **Mindset** | Review Progress Towards Your Goals | | |

THE 30-DAY PROGRAMME

| DAY 4 | DAY 5 | DAY 6 | DAY 7 |
|---|---|---|---|
| Daily Gratitude | Daily Gratitude | Daily Gratitude | Daily Gratitude |
| Rest | Resistance Session 2 | HIIT Session | Free Cardio |

| DAY 11 | DAY 12 | DAY 13 | DAY 14 |
|---|---|---|---|
| Daily Gratitude | Daily Gratitude | Daily Gratitude | Daily Gratitude |
| Rest | Resistance Session 2 | HIIT Session | Free Cardio |
| Vision Setting | | | |

| DAY 18 | DAY 19 | DAY 20 | DAY 21 |
|---|---|---|---|
| Daily Gratitude | Daily Gratitude | Daily Gratitude | Daily Gratitude |
| Rest | Resistance Session 2 | HIIT Session | Free Cardio |
| Mastering Habits | | | |

## WEEK 4

| AREA | DAY 22 | DAY 23 | DAY 24 |
|---|---|---|---|
| **Daily Practice** | Daily Gratitude | Daily Gratitude | Daily Gratitude |
| **Workouts** | Rest | Resistance Session 1 | HIIT Session |
| **Mindset** | Review Progress Towards Your Goals | | |

## 30-dayS IS JUST THE START. KEEP GOING…

| | | | |
|---|---|---|---|
| **Daily Practice** | Daily Gratitude | Daily Gratitude | Daily Gratitude |
| **Workouts** | Rest | Resistance Session 1 | HIIT Session |
| **Mindset** | Review Progress Towards Your Goals | | |

| **DAY 25** | **DAY 26** | **DAY 27** | **DAY 28** |
|---|---|---|---|
| Daily Gratitude | Daily Gratitude | Daily Gratitude | Daily Gratitude |
| Rest | Resistance Session 2 | HIIT Session | Free Cardio |
| Future Self | | | |

| | | | |
|---|---|---|---|
| Daily Gratitude | Daily Gratitude | Daily Gratitude | Daily Gratitude |
| Rest | Resistance Session 2 | HIIT Session | Free Cardio |

# Setting And Committing To Goals

*Before we get going on the next section you're going to commit to your goals.*

So, having read everything so far, what do you now want from your life? What have you been holding yourself back from that you deserve to go for? It doesn't have to be grand, but pick something.

I also want you to commit to your wellness goals now.

## Goals And Commitments

My life goal is (you'll do more specific work on this later in the programme):

_____

_____

_____

_____


My long term goals in terms of nutrition and fat loss are:

_____

_____

# THE 30-DAY PROGRAMME

For these four weeks I am committed to:

i. _____

ii. _____

iii. _____

My Current measurements: _____

Weight: _____

Body Fat: _____

Waist: _____

After 30-days

Weight: _____

Body Fat: _____

Waist: _____

My current Life Goal is:

_____

_____

_____

_____

After 30-days I have achieved:

_____

_____

_____

_____

_____

_____

# Mindset

*Mindset is the keystone to everything, so we're going to address that first. Throughout the 30-days of the programme we're going to introduce different elements to help train your mind to focus on your goals and help you feel both more present and more positive. Psychology and working on our mindset and emotional wellbeing is the most important part.*

So why does this matter? Well, the changes in hormones and neurotransmitters we experience during midlife have a direct impact on our emotions and thoughts, so they're already influencing our mood and thinking. Factor in the psychological fall-out from physiological changes, and you'll begin to understand why it's so important to get your mind as well as your body on side for true success.

There's a daily practice, and it's really important that you do this daily, then there will be a new mindset exercise for each week. Use these as often as you need to, they are the foundations for your success.

## Daily Gratitude Practice

First up is a daily practice, starting tomorrow. As soon as you're awake and before you let in the outside world by looking at your phone, turning on the TV or radio, find a few quiet minutes just to do the following:

Note down 3 things you were grateful for yesterday.

Note down 3 things you're grateful for generally.

Set an intention for today.

That's it. Really do feel the emotion of gratitude as you do this, we want to connect with our emotions, everything starts with an attitude of gratitude and you'll notice a positive shift in your energy once you've practised this a while.

This is really simple to do, you might want to buy a journal for this or you can just do it in your head.

Every morning reflect on 3 things you're grateful for from yesterday. These don't have to be big things, it could be as simple as the sun was shining and it made you smile.

Reflect on three things you're grateful for in general, and set an intention for the day.

Do this daily and see how your attitude to life shifts.

# Nutrition

*Here's how you're going to eat for the next 30-days. No calorie counting, no diet, no meal plan, just guiding principles to make it easy AND get results. Familiarise yourself with the principles then start planning your weeks eating in as much detail as you need for it to work for you.*

Often we'll go wrong when we're short on time, hungry and we haven't thought about what to eat. Planning ahead helps avoid this, also have a think about fall back, easy to prep, go to meals for when life gets in the way.

## Why You Shouldn't Focus On Losing Weight

DO NOT FOCUS ON LOSING WEIGHT! Focus on reducing BODY FAT. This is what we're aiming for. The scales aren't your friend, but the body fat monitors are. Muscle is denser than fat (therefore heavier) so you can actually weigh more (add lean muscle) but have reduced body fat and look much better. Go on how you feel and look. Forget your weight. I can't say this enough. And one last thing – don't check body fat more than every two weeks. It can lead to obsession, not progression.

If you want to check your body fat you can use callipers, which is cheap but fiddly or invest in some body composition scales. Tanita is a great brand and you can pick up a set for less than £30 at the time of writing.

On to diets. There are lots of crash diets out there, and as you all know – I am not a fan for a few reasons:

While they might work in the short term, they are rarely sustainable and chances are very high that you will put the weight (plus more) back on (one study found only 5% of people who crash diet keep the weight off).

They are rarely healthy. Often these diets deprive you of nutrients and macros you actually need to function.

Mentally and emotionally denial and guilt around food is not good. Food is essential for living and should be enjoyed, not something to have negative emotions around.

To safely drop body fat and keep it off, it's recommended to create a calorie deficit of around 500 to 600 calories per day. This can be done by cutting out 500 to 600 calories, additional exercise to burn 500 to 600 calories or a combination of both (this is what we recommend). With exercise this should equate to around 1 pound of fat loss per week. Remember to consider activity levels when calculating caloric intake and aim to consume the proper ratios of nutrients (more on this shortly).

Remember that cutting calories so that your training suffers can have the opposite effect to what you're intending (another reason to avoid crash diets). What we're aiming for is to lose body fat while maintaining muscle.

Cut too many calories and your body can go catabolic, meaning you burn muscle instead of fat. Your metabolism slows and you may even be more prone to putting fat on.

Ideally combine resistance and cardio exercise for both calorie burn and muscle tissue maintenance, whilst moderating your diet to hit that 500 calorie deficit. It's a gradual process, but one that reaps rewards.

Some of us may not want to lose weight, but actually want to add weight by building muscle mass. Again, the theory is simple, more exercise (especially resistance training to build muscle) and a calorie surplus.

If you're looking to bulk up it is important to consider and monitor your intensity of physical activity. We recommend increasing your calorie intake by around 300 calories per day, going up to 500 calories per day if you're not seeing gains after a couple of weeks. The make up of those calories in terms of the macro blend is important and we're going to look at that next.

Just before that though...

## A Word On Semaglutides

At the time of writing "weight loss" jabs are extremely popular. This family of drugs known as semaglutides come under the brand names Wegovy, Ozempic, Mounjaro and more.

Originally semaglutides were developed for diabetics, as they have a positive effect on insulin levels. A side effect was found to be a slowing of the emptying of the intestine resulting in more fullness and a hormonal effect resulting in less appetite.

There's no doubt that they are effective in helping weight loss, but here's the problem: it's weight loss not just fat loss. Some research suggests that the amount of muscle mass lost could be out of proportion to the fat tissue lost, particularly in midlife and older populations where we're already losing muscle. There could also be a negative effect on bone density.

A further issue is that with users relying on the drug's appetite suppression, there's no alteration of habits and behaviours – simply put, it's easy not to eat. But when users cease taking the drug many report not only putting their body fat back on, but having an even bigger appetite than before they started.

So, if you are going to go down this road, my caveat would be that you should also work on your habits around food, make sure you're getting adequate protein and be doing regular resistance training to support muscle maintenance and growth.

## Understanding Macros

Time to get a little more complex. Not all calories are created equal – we need to ensure the correct balance of types of calorie from the macronutrient types. For example a carbohydrate calorie is different to a protein calorie, which requires more energy to break down. There are three major macronutrients that the human body needs in order to function properly: carbohydrates, protein, and fats.

We're going to look at each in more detail in a moment, but for now we can understand what proportion of our daily calorific intake should come from each. This is important as the balance can affect hormonal levels that will impact fat loss and/or muscle building in the body. Depending on your aim the ratios are going to be different. To add bulk all the amounts will be higher as they account for a calorific surplus, to lose weight they'll be lower and fats and carbs will be in lower proportions.

So now we have the calories we should be getting from carbohydrates, fats and protein, depending on our body aim. As a broad rule proteins and carbs contain around 4 calories per gram, while fat contains 9 calories per gram. Of course within this come many variables according to type of fat, protein, carbohydrate.

## Carbohydrates

Carbs have gotten a bad name in recent years ("no carbs before Marbs") but they're essential for all bodily function. The confusion comes over the types of carbs out there. Here's a handy guide:

ALL carbohydrates are made of sugars but according to their composition we can classify them further:

Refined carbohydrates are all white flour products, white rice, most breakfast cereals, biscuits, cake, sugar in all its forms (man-made and processed). Removing the fibre means that the sugar (glucose) is easily absorbed leading to a rapid raise in blood sugar levels. The process means that 90% of the mineral and vitamin content is lost! Why is this bad? The metabolic process known as the Krebs cycle – that the body uses to turn carbohydrates into energy – relies on a host of nutrients to make this conversion efficiently e.g. B vitamins and magnesium – the very nutrients lost in the refining process!

Unrefined carbohydrates are plants in their natural state. These provide the cofactors needed for optimal usage of the Krebs cycle to manufacture enough energy.

Fibrous carbohydrates are veggies that grow above the ground, providing the body with a great source of vitamins, minerals and fibre so they do not raise our blood sugar levels as quickly. These fibres are also great for our gut health.

Starchy carbohydrates are root veggies and whole grains that have a high energy content and provide good amounts of nutrients. How they affect your blood sugar levels can vary.

Mixed carbohydrates (beans and pulses) contain a mixture of starch and fibre but they also provide more protein, which further slows down the rate sugar is released into our bloodstream providing a more steady stream of energy.

Fruit contains both glucose and fructose in varying amounts depending on the climate of where it is grown. Fructose is metabolised differently from glucose and does not raise your blood sugar levels in the same way however it can put a strain on your liver if eaten in too large a quantity.

Don't forget to count your vegetable intake as a carbohydrate source and aim for around 6 to 8 portions of vegetables a day. Ideally carbohydrates to maintain energy throughout the day need to be low GI (unrefined carbohydrates). However while generally speaking low GI is best, carbohydrates consumed post workout session (within 30 minutes) can be higher GI (e.g. sugary tropical fruits, fruit juices, honey, white rice cakes etc..) but should be eaten in combination with protein and/or fats to lessen insulin spikes.

## A Note On Processed And Ultra Processed Foods

These will mainly be carbohydrate based and you're looking to avoid foods with lots of chemical names on the label and anything that's gone through a lot of processes before it arrives to you. Aim to reduce your consumption of these as much as possible. Research shows that not only will we eat more of them, as they override our hormonal digestive responses, but that we're more likely to store them as body fat. They also have the potential to disrupt other hormonal pathways and negatively affect things like sleep and mood. They also have little nutritional value. Stick to fresh, whole and natural options, where you can.

## Fats

Fat has a bad rep, and perhaps rightly so, but in fact fat is essential for us. It's simply too much of the wrong kind of fat that is detrimental. Fat is made up of building blocks called fatty acids and these are classified as saturated, monounsaturated or polyunsaturated depending on their chemical structure.

## Saturated Fats

Saturated fats are the fats found in fatty meat cuts, dairy, and some palm and nut oils. Generally saturated fats are solid at room temperature. Too much saturated fat has been linked to raised cholesterol levels in the blood, which increases the risk of heart disease and stroke. There are two types of cholesterol in the body: HDL (good) cholesterol and LDL (bad) cholesterol. 'Bad' cholesterol can build up in our blood vessels and cause them to narrow, which in turn increases the risk of blood clots which can lead to heart attacks or strokes. 'Good' cholesterol retrieves the 'bad' cholesterol from the body and carries it to the liver so that too much doesn't build up in the bloodstream. Several studies have shown a high saturated fat intake to be linked with high cholesterol, and studies have shown that replacing saturated fat with unsaturated fat in the diet reduces blood cholesterol and lowers the risk of heart disease and stroke. Try to limit the amount of saturated fat in your diet as much as possible.

## Trans Fats

Trans fats are found naturally in small amounts in meat and dairy products, but much larger amounts are made in the production of partially hydrogenated vegetable oils. Until fairly recently this was used a lot in various spreads, baked products and more, but it's use has been cut back due to health concerns. To lower trans fat intake, avoid processed foods as much as possible.

## Unsaturated Fats

The good ones! Unsaturated fats contain a higher proportion of unsaturated fatty acids and are usually liquid at room temperature. Monounsaturated and polyunsaturated fats help to maintain healthy cholesterol levels and are found in vegetable oils such as olive, rapeseed and sunflower oils, avocados, nuts and seeds.

Polyunsaturated fats provide us with essential fatty acids like omega 3 which are important for health.

Try to get as much of your fat macros from unsaturated fats as possible. Think oily fish (e.g. mackerel, salmon and sardines) and in smaller amounts in sunflower oil, flax, linseed oil and walnuts. Omega 3 fatty acids are associated with good heart health as they can help to prevent blood clotting and regulate heart rhythm. In order to get the benefits from these fatty acids we should all aim to eat at least one portion of oily fish per week.

Fat is not just an efficient and plentiful energy source, it also provides cell membrane fluidity allowing nutrients to flow in and out of the cells that means our body can function at a more efficient rate. Omega 3 also reduces inflammation and has been shown to enhance post-training recovery.

Medium chain fatty acids such as those found in coconut oil and omega 3 speed up the metabolism and have been shown effective in losing weight. They also aid concentration and energy, as the brain is the richest source of fatty acids.

Medium chain fatty acids found in coconut oil are readily converted into energy by the liver rather than being stored as fat and have been shown to have a positive impact on body composition when used regularly (1–2 tablespoons a day). However coconut oil is still a saturated fat so don't over use it.

## Protein

Protein is the building block of muscle. Protein is utilised in the body to make and repair muscle tissue. We actually build muscle at rest, not when lifting: when we over stimulate the muscle by lifting a heavy weight or repeated use, we actually create micro tears in the muscle tissue.

When we're at rest these tears repair, in effect scarring and this is what increases the muscle size and strength (they repair stronger). For the muscle to grow (i.e. repair effectively) we need protein as the building block. This is also why rest days from training are important. If you were to hit the same muscle day after day with no rest, it would never get the chance to repair and would fatigue – which we know as overtraining.

Protein is found in lean red meats, white meats (poultry, fish) and to a slightly lesser extent in seeds, nuts, pulses and dairy. You will have already worked out your macros but as a rule of thumb if you're looking to increase muscle mass, then between 1–2g of protein per kilogram of bodyweight is recommended.

To ensure you get enough protein, protein shakes are a really efficient and easy way to boost intake. Added bonus is that they will also contain BCAAs (see below). When choosing a shake try to get one without any chemical additives. Most studies suggest that the body can't effectively absorb and utilise more than around 30g of protein in one go, so spread your protein intake through the day.

## Other Nutrient Considerations

Those are the macros dealt with, within those we want to ensure the micronutrients are present. In practice following a balanced diet of unrefined food will deliver you the nutrient mix you need, however, here are a few extra pointers to look out for:

## Magnesium

Is the magic mineral we could all do with more of. It helps relax the mind and the body (muscles) but also gives us energy so it's important to get sufficient levels when regularly exercising. Magnesium rich foods are seaweeds, nuts, seeds and DGLV (dark green leafy vegetables) such as spinach, kale, rocket, watercress, parsley, chard, broccoli and savoy cabbage. Epsom bath salts are magnesium sulphate and are an effective way to increase your levels of magnesium. A large mug in a hot bath for 15–30 minutes, three times a week can be very beneficial as magnesium is well absorbed through the skin. You can also find magnesium oils to rub into the skin.

## Zinc

Plays a key role in hormonal health and in supporting our immune system. We can ingest it from red meat and nuts but it can be worth supplementing with to boost levels.

## Antioxidants

Free radical formation is a natural by-product of metabolic processes. In basic terms, when we stress the body we produce harmful free radicals, for instance during exercise the oxidative load on the body increases and more free radicals are produced. If this system is not suitably balanced by antioxidant protection, inflammation or tissue degradation can occur. Therefore it is important to eat lots of antioxidant rich dark green leafy vegetables, berries and some nuts and seeds.

## Vitamin C

Is a water soluble vitamin and therefore can leech from the body with sweating and exercise. It also plays a role in muscle tissue development, so consider vitamin C supplementation. It's also great for the immune system.

## Vitamin D

Is actually a steroid hormone not a vitamin! We synthesise it ourselves through exposure to sunlight, rather than ingesting it, meaning that if we don't live somewhere sunny and/or spend a lot of time indoors, levels can be low. Vitamin D plays a role in supporting our hormonal health and our immune system, so if you're not getting much outside exposure to sunlight this can be worth supplementing.

## Fibre

Keeps everything moving. It's important to consume enough leafy greens, beans and pulses, but sometimes on a protein rich diet you may require a little extra. Our gut biomes (responsible for producing neurotransmitters which affect mood) love fibre to feed off (pre-biotic), which is another great reason to ensure you have enough in your diet.

## Pro-biotics

Are also great for our gut health, think live yogurts and fermented food, but you might find it easier to take a pro-biotic supplement.

## Branch Chain Amino Acids (BCAAs)

Are the essential building blocks of muscle. Not really needed if your goal is weight loss, but if you're aiming to add muscle and/or your physical activity level is intense, consider supplementing with these. Protein powder has BCAAs in, so if you have that you don't need a separate BCAA as well.

## H2O

Our bodies are around half to two thirds water, so staying properly hydrated is not only key for effective physical function, but mental clarity and function too. I recommend at least 1.5 litres of water a day, more if training intensively and/or in hot or humid conditions where you sweat more.

## Putting It All Together

To summarise and give you a very basic principle for nutrition, I believe that 'from field or sea to table, in as few steps as possible', will provide you with a healthy, varied, and delicious diet.

As a general rule of thumb, the more steps the item on your plate has been through before it got there, probably the worse it is for you. So think less pre-bought breaded chicken and oven chips and more grilled fish served on a bed of salad, stir fried chicken with fresh vegetables, a lean steak grilled with a big serving of fresh spinach and so on.

My other motto is 'everything in moderation'. Knowing what are bad food choices and moderating them will reap dividends, but at the same time, don't deny yourself the occasional treat.

You now have the information, on the following pages you'll find the principles you need to start winning at nutrition, using simple methodology and hand sizes for portions.

Always give a change in eating and exercise at least two weeks to see any results – experiment, have fun with it and find what works for you.

You'll see on the next few pages a guide to macro sizes using your hand, which is a really simple way to stay on track, along with a guide to what your plate should look like in macro terms.

Remember, you're just looking to get this broadly right across the day, please don't obsess about it.

Herbs, spices and low calorie sauces are great ways to liven up food and keep it interesting, so include those as much as you like.

Okay, here's the hand measuring system for food:

Protein: Two palm sized portions of lean protein at every meal

Fats: Two thumb sized portions at every meal

Carbohydrates: Two cupped palm sized portions for breakfast and lunch, none at dinner

Vegetables: Two fist sized portions at every meal

THE 30-DAY PROGRAMME

**PORTION CONTROL PER MEAL**
(based on 3 meals per day)

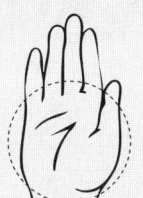

**1 PALM SIZE** PORTION OF **LEAN PROTEIN** AT EVERY MEAL FOR **WOMEN**

**2 PALM SIZE** PORTION OF **LEAN PROTEIN** AT EVERY MEAL FOR **MEN**

Palm sized portion of lean protein, both in width and thickness with every meal. Choose protein dense foods such as meat, fish, dairy and beans.

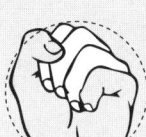

**1 FIST SIZED** PORTION OF **VEGETABLES** AT EVERY MEAL FOR **WOMEN**

**2 FIST SIZED** PORTION OF **VEGETABLES** AT EVERY MEAL FOR **MEN**

Closed fist sized portion of vegetables with every meal. Vegetables such as broccoli, spinach, carrots, peppers, mushrooms, etc..

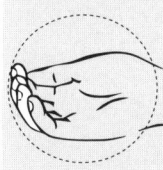

**1 CUPPED SIZE** PORTION OF LOW GI **CARBOHYDRATES** FOR **WOMEN** – 2 MEALS (BREAKFAST AND LUNCH)

**1 CUPPED SIZE** PORTION OF LOW GI **CARBOHYDRATES** FOR **MEN** – 2–3 MEALS

Eat cupped handful of carbohydrate dense foods like grains and starches with breakfast and lunch e.g. oats, brown rice, quinoa. If you're looking to loose body fat, front load your carbs in the first half of the day and aim not to have any after 4pm. For example – breakfast and lunch but not dinner.

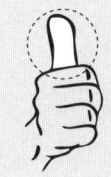

**1 THUMB SIZE** PORTION OF HEALTHY **FATS** AT EVERY MEAL FOR **WOMEN**

**2 THUMB SIZE** PORTION OF HEALTHY **FATS** AT EVERY MEAL FOR **MEN**

Thumb sized portion of healthy fats with every meal. Include fat dense foods such as nuts, seed, oils, avocado, nut butter etc..

Next up we have the macro ratio as it would look on a plate. Rethink your breakfast to ensure you're getting enough protein at that meal, a protein based smoothie is a great way to go (scoop of protein powder, 400ml water, handful of berries, half to three quarter cup of oats, dash of cinnamon). Keep snacks to a minimum and go for high protein snacks like a small amount of nuts, nut butter or yogurt with protein powder and you can eat 1 to 2 pieces of fruit a day, but not in the evening.

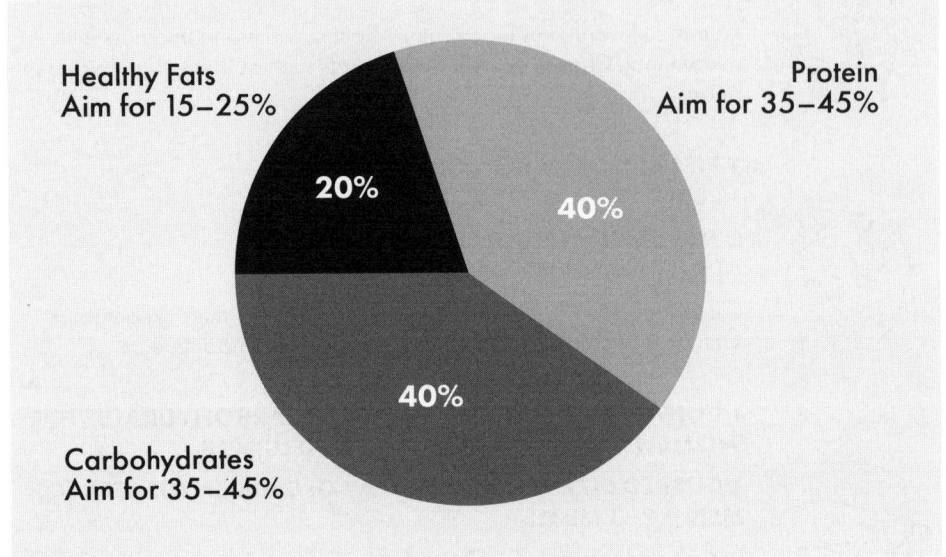

# THE 30-DAY PROGRAMME

Here are some food examples for each macro (not exhaustive). Consider the quality of your food and aim to eat like this 80% of the time and how you want the other 20%.

**Protein Options** (2 Palm Size Portions)

| MEAT PROTEIN | SEAFOOD PROTEIN | OTHER PROTEIN |
|---|---|---|
| Lean beef steak | White Fish (cod, haddock etc.) | Eggs |
| Lean beef mince | Oily fish (salmon, mackerel etc.) | Quorn |
| Lean cuts of beef | Tuna | Tofu |
| Chicken | Prawns | Beans |
| Turkey | Smoked fish (salmon, trout) | Lentils |
| Pork Chops | | |
| Gammon Steak | | |
| Ham | | |
| Bacon | | |

**Fats Options** (2 Thumb Size Portions)

| NUTS AND SEEDS | OILS | OTHER |
|---|---|---|
| All nuts | Olive oil | Natural cheeses |
| Sunflower seeds | Coconut oil (extra virgin) | Cow's milk |
| Pumpkin seeds | Avocado | Coconut milk |
| Linseed | Flaxseed | Almond milk |
| Chia seeds | | Avocado |
| Sesame seeds | | |
| Nut butters (no salt, sugar or oil) | | |

**Carbohydrate Options** (2 Cupped Palm Size Portions Breakfast and Lunch Only)

| FRUITS | STARCHY (KEEP TO A MINIMUM) |
|---|---|
| Berries (all types) | Potato |
| Apples | Sweet potato |
| Tomato | Squashes |
| Olives | Rice (all types) |
| Banana (half only) | Quinoa |
| | Wholemeal bread |
| | Sourdough bread |
| | Wholemeal pittas |
| | Wraps |

**Vegetables** (2 Fist Size Portions)

### VEGETABLES

Artichoke

Asparagus

Aubergine

Bean sprouts

Broccoli

Brussel sprouts

Cabbage

Cauliflower

Carrots

Celery

Courgette

Tomato

Leafy greens (lettuce/leaves)

Leeks

Mushrooms

Onions

Peas in pod

Spinach

Peppers

Radishes

# Movement

*Included in this book is a four week movement programme combining short HIIT sessions and resistance training sessions you can do with water bottles, or dumbbells if you have them.*

This programme is designed for the novice, so by all means if you have a resistance programme you already follow, or a preferred form of HIIT do that.

The key things are:

For resistance training hit each muscle group twice a week with at least 48 hours recovery before hitting it again.

Ensure progression – so either a higher weight or more reps as you get stronger.

Do your HIIT on a separate day to your resistance training.

If possible do your HIIT fasted first thing to help reduce body fat and give you an endorphin boost for the day. Do your resistance training fuelled.

Remember to always warm up before a workout and cool down and stretch afterwards.

If you're unsure of any of the moves, check online for the correct form.

Perform HIIT on Monday and Thursday, with a steady state cardio such as a gentle run, swim, row or bike ride at the weekend.

Perform resistance on Tuesday and Friday.

Wednesday is a rest day.

# HIIT

One of the reasons we hear a lot for people not exercising is a lack of time. Another common one is a lack of knowledge, so we thought we'd give you a brief introduction to HIIT – High Intensity Interval Training.

It's got a great name, but what is it? Simply put HIIT involves exercising as hard as you can for brief periods of time (the high intensity bit) with rest pauses which allow your heart rate to go down slightly (the interval part).

So for example, you might sprint for 20 seconds and then rest for 10 seconds, before sprinting again.

There are many ways you can do it, perhaps the simplest is the Tabata. The Tabata came out of research in Japan looking at the optimum intervals and timings for HIIT, and the result was a 4 minute block of 20 seconds work, with 10 seconds rest.

I love Tabatas because it's simple, effective and you can download Tabata timers for free on all app stores (just search for Tabata).

Now four minutes might not seem like long, but if you're going hard (and you should be) you will find it challenging. As your fitness increases you can add two or three Tabata's together, and if you're doing three, that's only 12 minutes of exercise but you will get results.

Now the key for HIIT is to go as hard as you can during those 20 seconds of work, you want to get out of breath and create what we call an oxygen debt.

You can do HIIT on a bike or rower, sprinting then resting. The way we like to coach our clients to do it is to simply pair two different bodyweight exercises and alternate them. For example squat jumps and press ups. Just repeat through the sequence alternating them.

HIIT is effective because the interval effect and resulting rise and fall in heart rate, coupled with oxygen debt spikes the body's metabolism. What this means in practice is that not only is your cardiovascular fitness improving, but after a HIIT session you'll carry on burning calories at a higher rate for around 24 hours.

In short, the benefits are multiple: it is simple and quick to do, gives you cardiovascular and calorie burning results, and it can be done anywhere – you just need space to move.

You can download free Tabata timers, and I'd like you to start with two Tabatas back to back, where you pair two cardio exercises from the list below (check online if you're unsure on any of the moves). As you get fitter, add a third, then fourth Tabata.

## The Moves

Pair two moves for each 4 minute Tabata:

- Squat or Squat Jumps
- Star Jumps
- Lunges or Lunge Jumps
- Press Ups
- Running on the spot
- Burpees
- Mountain Climbers
- Skipping/Air Skips
- Froggers
- Bum Kicks
- Side Lunges
- Tuck Jumps
- Standing Knee to Elbow
- Broad Jumps

## Squat Or Squat Jumps

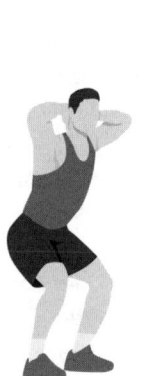
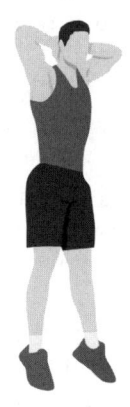

## Star Jumps

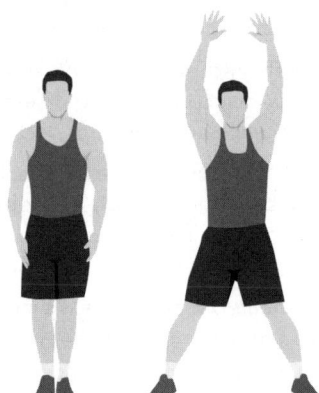

## Lunges Or Lunge Jumps

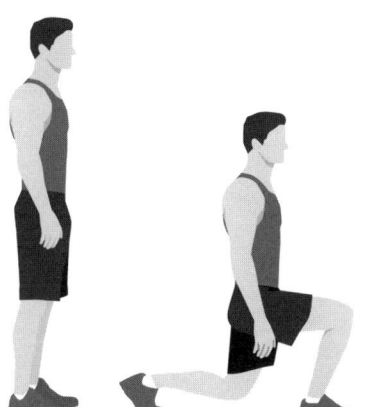

## Press Ups

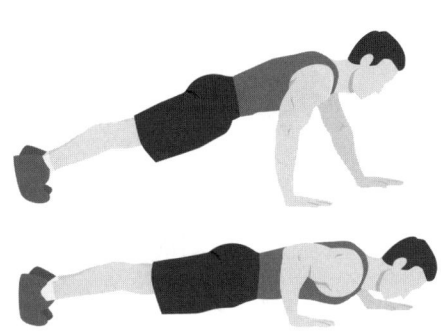

## Running On The Spot

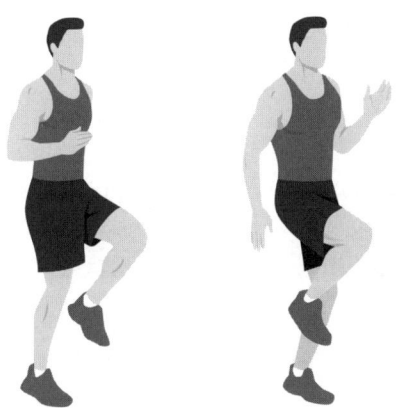

## Burpees

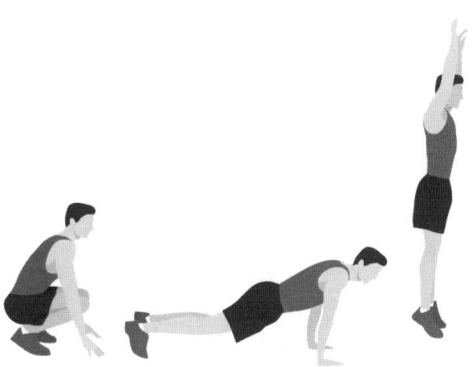

## Mountain Climbers

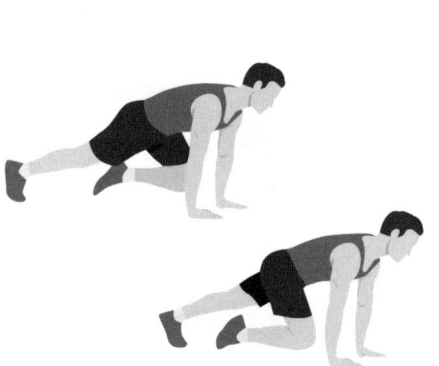

## Skipping / Air Skips

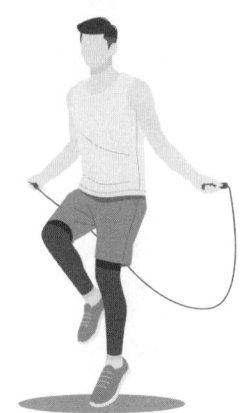

## Froggers

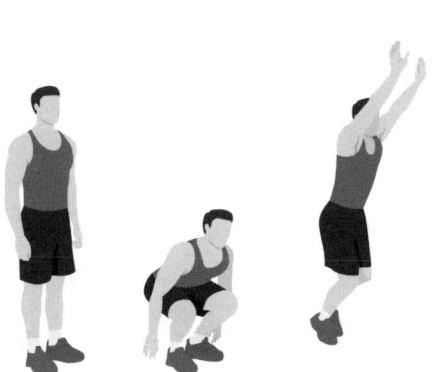

## Bum Kicks

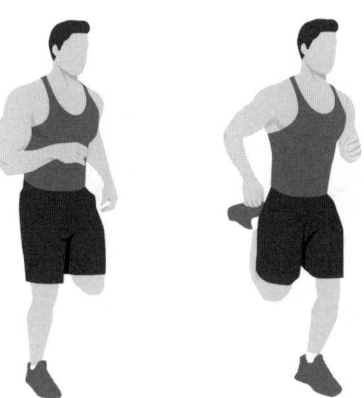

THE 30-DAY PROGRAMME

## Side Lunges

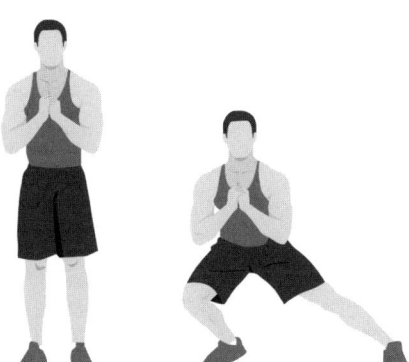

## Tuck Jumps

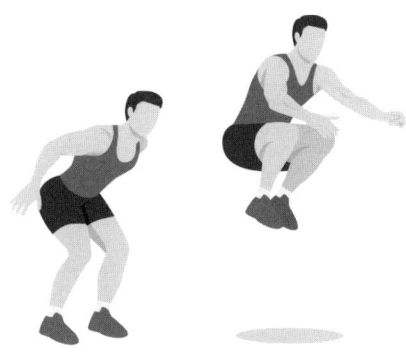

## Plank Jacks

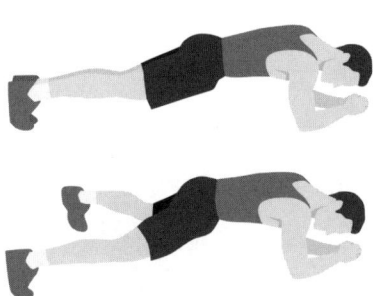

## Crunches

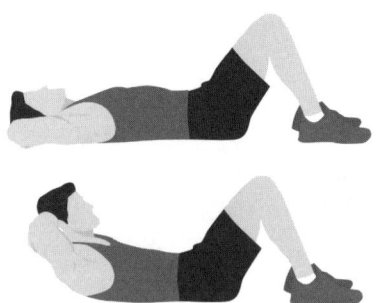

## Resistance

Use dumbbells and bodyweight for your resistance sessions below. Go back to back so from Dumbbell Squat to Weighted Step Back Lunge, to Squat Jumps and so on until you hit the end of the circuit.

To begin with do one round, you should be doing two rounds with a two minute rest between rounds by week two, and aim for three rounds in week three and four rounds in week four.

If you start to find the weight you're using easy to finish the final round with, then increase it slightly next time around.

If you don't have dumbbells you can use filled water bottles as weights.

### Dbell Squat OR Goblet Squat

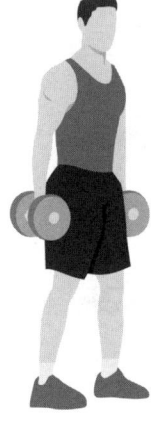
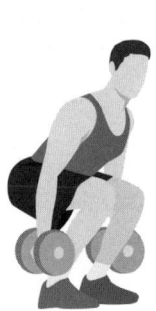

### Weighted Step Back Lunge

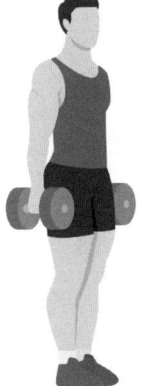
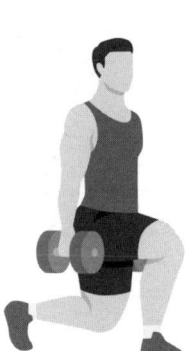

## THE 30-DAY PROGRAMME

## Squat Or Squat Jumps

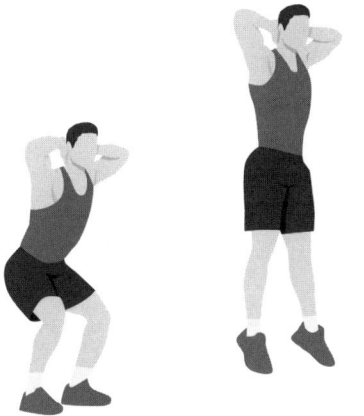

## Press Ups

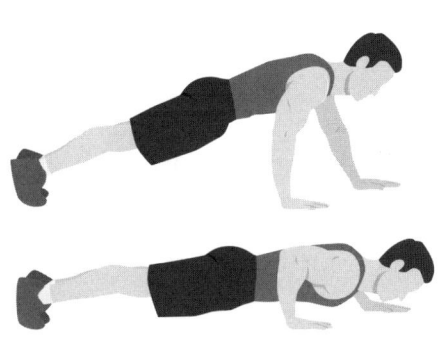

## Dbell Plank Row

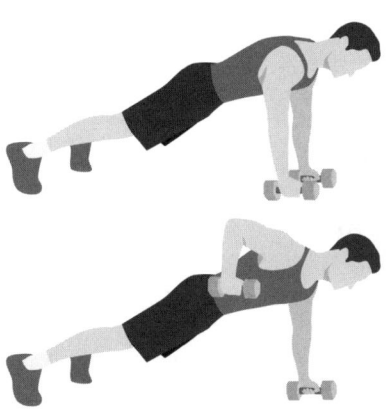

## Bent Over Back Flies

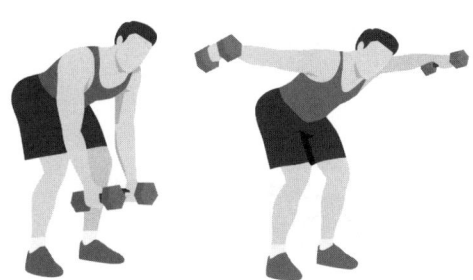

## Dbell Shoulder Press

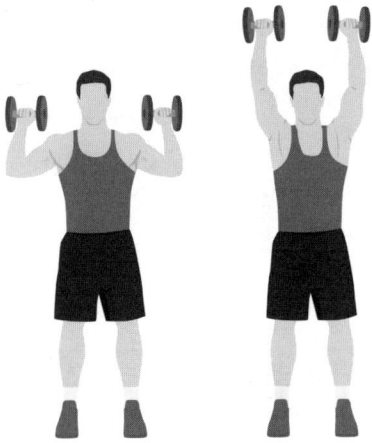

## Hammer Curls

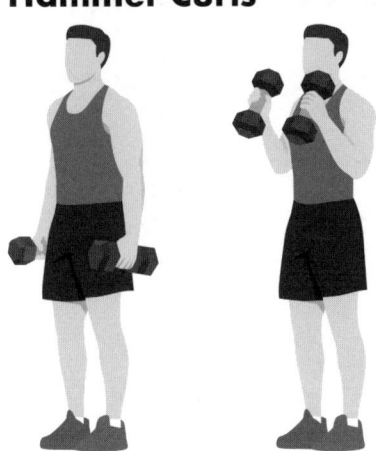

## Close Hands Press Up

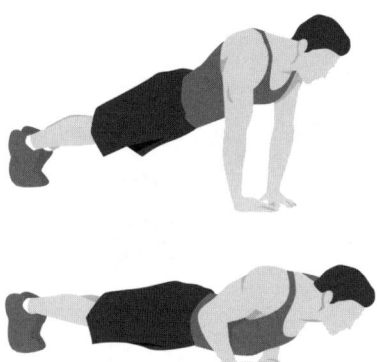

## Steering Wheels

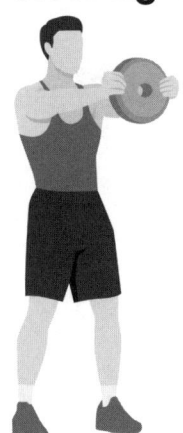

## Lunges Or Lunge Jumps

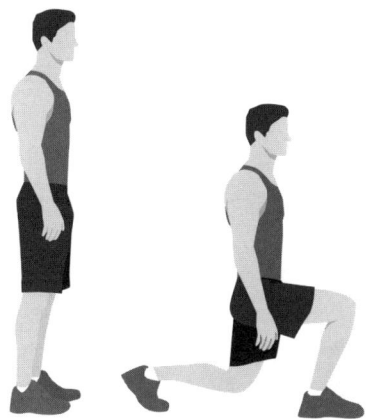

## Dbell Upright Row

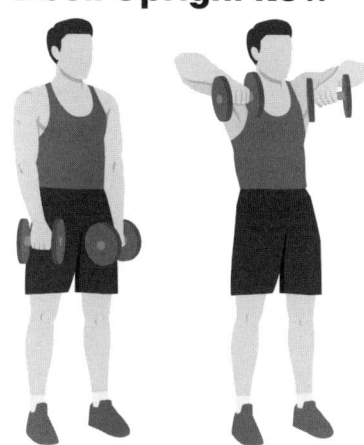

## Bent Over Dbell Row

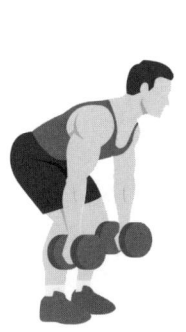
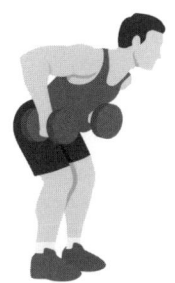

## Lat Raises

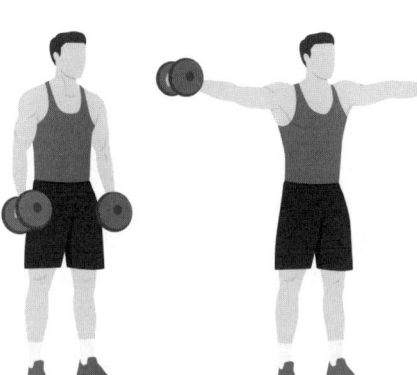

## Dbell Curls

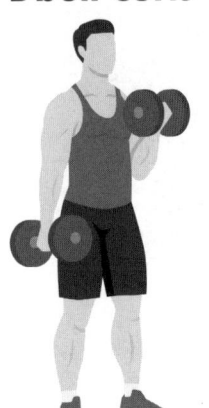

## Tricep Dips (off low table)

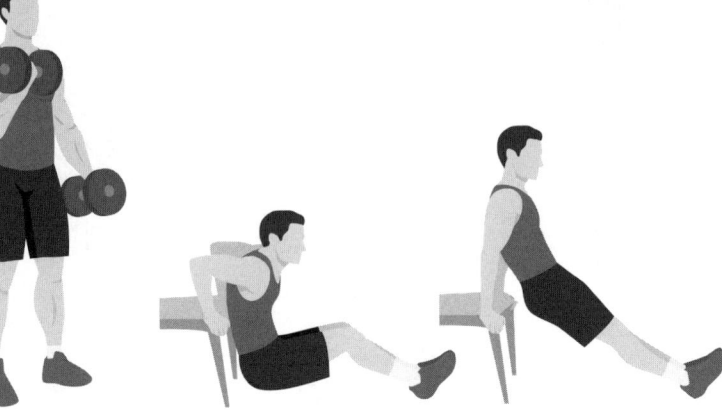

## Front Raises

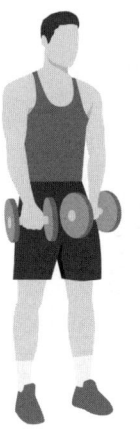
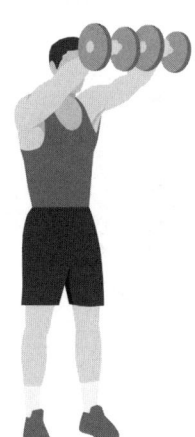

THE 30-DAY PROGRAMME

## Resistance Session 1

| Exercise | Body part / Muscle | WEIGHT | | | |
|---|---|---|---|---|---|
| | | Week 1 | Week 2 | Week 3 | Week 4 |
| Dbell Squat OR Goblet Squat | Legs/Quads | | | | |
| Weighted Step Back Lunge | Legs/Glutes/Hamstrings | | | | |
| Squat Jumps (no weight) | Chest | | | | |
| Press Ups | Chest | | | | |
| Dbell Plank Row | Back | | | | |
| Bent Over Back Flies | Back | | | | |
| Dbell Shoulder Press | Shoulders | | | | |
| Hammer Curls | Biceps | | | | |
| Close Hands Press Up | Triceps | | | | |
| Steering Wheels | Shoulders | | | | |

## Resistance Session 2

| Exercise | Body part / Muscle | WEIGHT | | | |
|---|---|---|---|---|---|
| | | Week 1 | Week 2 | Week 3 | Week 4 |
| Dbell Squat OR Goblet Squat | Legs/Quads | | | | |
| Weighted Step Back Lunge | Legs/Glutes/Hamstrings | | | | |
| Lunge Jumps (no weight) | Chest | | | | |
| Press Ups | Chest | | | | |
| Dbell Upright Row | Shoulders | | | | |
| Bent Over Dbell Row | Back | | | | |
| Lat Raises | Shoulders | | | | |
| Dbell Curls | Biceps | | | | |
| Tricep Dips (off low table) | Triceps | | | | |
| Front Raises | Shoulders | | | | |

# Week 1:
## Life Equilibrium

*This is your starting point and the first thing we need to do is know where we're starting from. This week along with your daily gratitude practice, regular exercise and abiding by your new nutrition principles, we're going to look at your life balance and start moving you to the right equilibrium for you and your goals.*

**Remember Your Goals And Stay Resolute**

| REMINDER: | YOUR WEEK LOOKS LIKE THIS EXERCISE WISE: |
|---|---|
| Monday: | HIIT (20–25 minutes) |
| Tuesday: | Resistance Training (30–45 minutes) |
| Wednesday: | Rest |
| Thursday: | HIIT (20–25 minutes) |
| Friday: | Resistance Training (30–45 minutes) |
| Saturday: | Steady State Cardio (45–90 minutes) |
| Sunday: | Rest |

Energy goes where intention flows. Or looking at it another way, which plants are you watering and caring for and which have been left in a dark corner unloved? Which do you think will be flourishing?

Are you spending all your time immersed in work so your relationships are suffering? Are you neglecting your own personal growth in favour of chasing financial gain?

Is there a mismatch in where you're expending your energy and what you actually want from life? Sometimes we want something to change, but we don't realise we're actually neglecting it by directing our time and energy elsewhere.

We're all given the same amount of time in a day. And whatever you're focusing on during that time, that's where you're going to see progress.

It really is as simple as that.

So...

Complete the following chart to see where the energy gap is, where you are out of equilibrium.

Assess with a number between 1–10 how much time and energy you're currently spending in each area. 1 meaning no time, 10 meaning a lot.

Next, go to the column that says "Optimal". Write down what would be the optimal time spent in each area, to live the life that you want? This is where you'd want your energy to be in your ideal life.

> *"Energy goes where intention flows. Or looking at it another way, which plants are you watering and caring for and which have been left in a dark corner unloved? Which do you think will be flourishing?"*

|  | Currently | Optimal |
|---|---|---|
| Work/Finance |  |  |
| Self/Growth |  |  |
| Relationships |  |  |
| Body/Health |  |  |

You should be spending more time in areas where you want to see more results. Are you? Or are you expanding energy in things that seem important now but aren't really part of your bigger purpose?

Also, don't fool yourself by thinking you can increase your score in every area – remember that we all only have 24 hours in a day.

How balanced is your life equilibrium, and now you know, what are you doing to do about it?

## Example

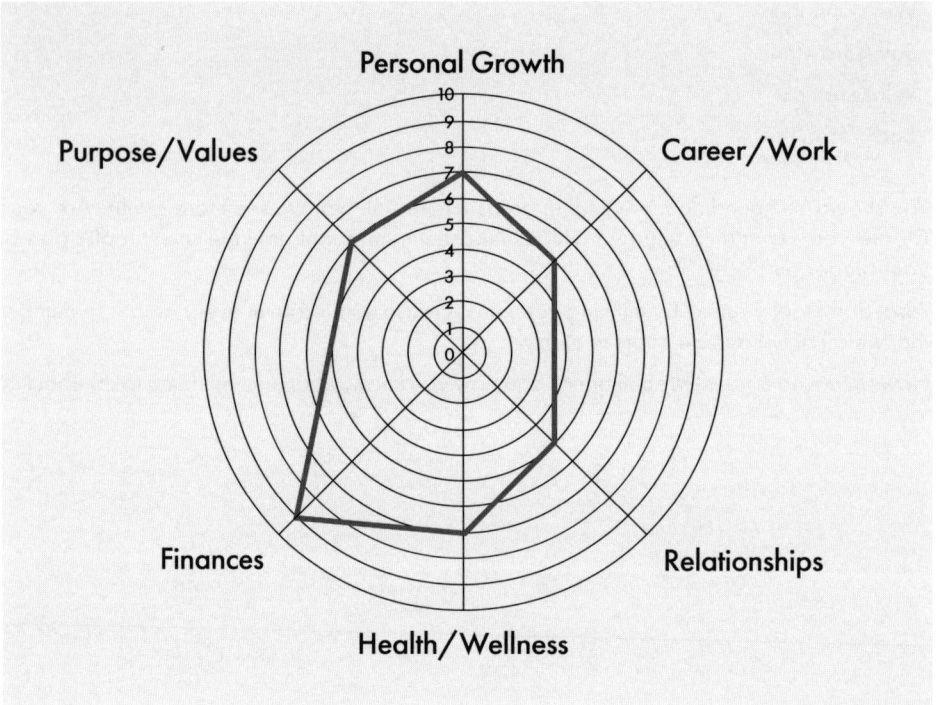

## Your Chart

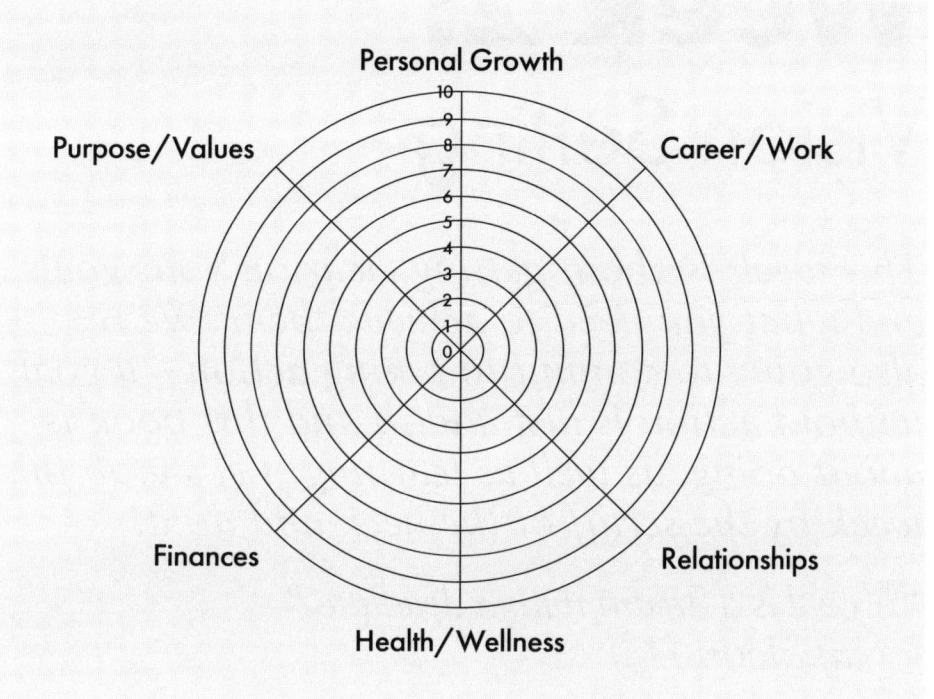

# Week 2:
## Vision Setting

*This week is about getting clear on your goals and what you need to achieve them. We're also going to commit to taking action – a goal without action is just a wish and this book is about doing, as well as learning. Let's grab this week by the scruff of the neck and do it!*

*"A goal is a dream with a deadline."*
*– Napoleon Hill*

### Remember Your Goals And Stay Resolute

| REMINDER: | YOUR WEEK LOOKS LIKE THIS EXERCISE WISE: |
|---|---|
| Monday: | HIIT (20–25 minutes) |
| Tuesday: | Resistance Training (30–45 minutes) |
| Wednesday: | Rest |
| Thursday: | HIIT (20–25 minutes) |
| Friday: | Resistance Training (30–45 minutes) |
| Saturday: | Steady state cardio (45–90 minutes) |
| Sunday: | Rest |

When we dream big we get inspired, so don't limit yourself, what do you really want? We're going to apply some filters later. This process is about figuring out how we bring these goals to life and creating an action plan.

Note that research shows we're 30% more likely to achieve our goals when we write them down, you'll be well on the way.

# TASK 1

Write down 3 goals you'd like to achieve in the next year.

They can be anything around your physical, mental and emotional wellbeing.

Or any other goal you might have.

Allow yourself to think BIG. Don't let fear hold you back, don't restrict your goals by judging them.

# TASK 2

Be specific.

Very often the reason we 'fail' at certain goals is because we've put absolutely no parameters around it.

We need detail in order to 'buy into' the vision – so it feels good....

Use the following format to create a statement around your goal:

**S**pecific

**M**easurable

**A**chievable

**R**ealistic/Relevant (To Me)

**T**ime Bound

EXAMPLE

I will lose 12lbs of weight in the next 8 weeks by looking after my nutrition and moving my body daily to create a calorie deficit.

You get the idea, "I want to lose weight" is not a goal it's a wish. Breaking any goal down using SMART gives you the steps to achieve it and the foundation of a plan. Now write yours down:

## TASK 3

Engage Emotion – The "Why".

Start asking yourself some of these questions below for each goal....

Why do I want this?

Why is it so important to me?

Why is it important I do something about this now?

How will my life look different?

How will it make me feel?

# TASK 4

Dig Deeper.

What are some of the stumbling blocks I might encounter towards achieving my goal?

Start with the external:

Which ones do I have control over?

What is my plan when these stumbling blocks come up?

What will I do to ensure they don't derail me?

# TASK 5

Take Action.

Remember, a goal without action is just a wish! The magic ingredient between goals and outcomes is action.

What 3 things can you commit to DOING in the next 2 weeks that will take you towards your most important goal? Write them down:

# Week 3:
# Habit Shift

*Mastering our habits will allow us to move towards our goals more easily. It sets us up for a lifetime of the behaviours we need in order to be successful at taking positive action. So, let's get on top of those unhelpful habits and create our new helpful habits for long term success.*

*"We are what we repeatedly do. Excellence, then, is not an act, but a habit." – Will Durant*

### Remember Your Goals And Stay Resolute

| REMINDER: | YOUR WEEK LOOKS LIKE THIS EXERCISE WISE: |
|---|---|
| Monday: | HIIT (20–25 minutes) |
| Tuesday: | Resistance Training (30–45 minutes) |
| Wednesday: | Rest |
| Thursday: | HIIT (20–25 minutes) |
| Friday: | Resistance Training (30–45 minutes) |
| Saturday: | Steady state cardio (45–90 minutes) |
| Sunday: | Rest |

Habits are amazing things, they allow us to repeat actions daily, without even really thinking consciously about them. Think about brushing your teeth, or like I mentioned earlier, about learning to drive a car – remember how hard that was when you first sat in the driver's seat – the wheel, the pedals, the mirrors, the indicator stalks... now (if you drive) you can hop into a car and drive without really thinking. That's the power of habits.

However sometimes habits are not helpful, the good news is, we can change them. When we practise a habit day after day it becomes stronger, in fact it builds and strengthens a neural pathway in our brain to make the behaviour easier for us.

Knowing that, we can also use that to help change unhelpful habits that aren't aligned with our goal.

What I'd like you to do is make a list of any unhelpful habits you currently have that are going to hinder you achieving your goals. I'd recommend no more than five.

Note down a few habits you think may hinder you achieving your goal:

Now note down habits that you may need to foster in order to achieve your goal, again go for no more than five:

Great, now pick the one habit that is going to have the biggest positive impact on helping you achieve your goal and commit to changing one of those in the next few weeks. Don't try to change more than one at a time.

Check in with yourself:

Is it achievable?

Do you genuinely believe that you can build this habit? Have you got the time in your day and do you really want to build it?

Is it sustainable?

Do you believe that you can stick to this routine over a long time without running out of energy or money or other resources?

Is it appealing?

Is it something that resonates with you? If it's not appealing, go back and create a new habit that is appealing, you have to want it.

Finally, keep it simple! Go for a simple habit and make it clear to yourself what you're going to do to help build it.

Okay, so now onto the practical side.

A habit has three parts:

the **trigger or cue** that initiates the **behaviour**, then the **reward**.

For example, when I shut my laptop at the end of the day (trigger), I go to the cupboard to get a biscuit (behaviour) and enjoy eating it (reward).

So we want to address those three parts for our new habit. We want to create what we call implementation intentions.

First up, create a trigger for yourself – for example, when I get up (trigger)...

Then a behaviour – this is what is taking you towards your goal – I find a quiet space with my notebook and do my gratitude list (behaviour)...

Then a reward – once I have done that I make myself a delicious cup of coffee (reward).

If we can set a trigger that's at the same time, so much the better, our subconscious loves routine and will help wire it in faster.

Make the reward something you'll enjoy at that time and genuinely look forward to.

As a bonus to help you I want you to think of a pattern interrupt when you're tempted by your old unhelpful habit. Pattern interrupt is a term from hypnosis and Neuro Linguistic Programming where we break the thought pattern to bring awareness and establish a new pattern. For example, snapping an elastic band on your wrist or clicking your fingers...

Also research shows that if we become aware of the cue/trigger and can resist the behaviour for 5 seconds or longer, the drive to do the behaviour rapidly diminishes.

So do the above and mentally state the new helpful habit and how it's going to both reward you and benefit you, to help keep you focused.

Then practise, practise, practise. Consistency is key here to shift those old patterns to new ones.

# Week 4:
## Future Self

*This final week is about really engaging your mind to create the future you desire. I want you to remember that this 4 week programme is just a foundation. You can, and should, use these skills consistently after the 4 weeks to help maintain your forward progress. Remember to check in on your goals, celebrate wins, course correct where you need to and set new ones as your life evolves.*

### Always, Remember Your Goals And Stay Resolute

| REMINDER: | YOUR WEEK LOOKS LIKE THIS EXERCISE WISE: |
|---|---|
| Monday: | HIIT (20–25 minutes) |
| Tuesday: | Resistance Training (30–45 minutes) |
| Wednesday: | Rest |
| Thursday: | HIIT (20–25 minutes) |
| Friday: | Resistance Training (30–45 minutes) |
| Saturday: | Steady state cardio (45–90 minutes) |
| Sunday: | Rest |

## A Letter To Your Future Self

We talked about the power of future rehearsal, and one way you can utilise your imagination to align with your goals is to write a letter from your future self of one year from now, back to your present day self.

This is a form of visualisation and can also help get us really clear on what we want, or don't want and prime our subconscious for change.

It can be a very powerful exercise, so please take your time. See what comes up for you.

It doesn't need to be long, I'd recommend 5 to 6 paragraphs.

I'd like you to in the first paragraph thank your present self for not giving up on you, and helping you achieve all that you have achieved in the last 12 months.

In the second paragraph, snapshot your current situation – don't spend too long on this part, but get the essentials down.

For the rest of the letter I'd like you to really get into the emotion of what it feels like to have achieved what you have achieved, use rich language and engage as many emotions and senses as you can.

Here are some ideas:

- What does your life look like now and how do you feel?
- What do you spend most of your time doing, how does it feel?
- What is currently important to you?
- Who do you hang out with and what are those relationships like?
- What have you achieved in the last 12 months and what are you focusing on now?
- How does it feel to have achieved these things?
- How's your energy and health?
- Your finances?
- Your life balance?
- What do you drive?
- Where do you live?
- Who are you, 1 year from now?

For the final paragraph thank your present self again.

Save the letter and look at it regularly to remind yourself of your goals. It's great to formally review this every three months to track your progress and see if any of your goals have shifted. Enjoy!

## Accountability

The final thing we're going to talk about is accountability. Now, we can be accountable to ourselves, which is a form of discipline, but the research shows that when we are accountable to others, we're much more likely to succeed at our goals.

It's tough going it alone, so get some support. That might mean joining an online community where everyone is on a similar journey (like our own fab free Facebook community The Midlife Mentors community – search for it and ask to join).

It might mean getting a buddy you work on your goals with, joining some sort of group mastermind, or working with a coach or mentor.

Personally every time I want to level up I work with coaches for the particular area or goal I'm focusing on. That can mean I'm working with anything from one to six coaches at a time.

I made the mistake once of thinking I could maintain momentum and figure everything out on my own, and guess what? I wasn't accountable, everything suffered!

If you'd like to work with me, then reach out, there's contact info in the Next Steps section, but do reach out and find some support, be that online, real life, a PT or a friend...

It's always great to have someone with experience in your corner cheering you on, and it not only means you get there faster, but that you have more fun doing it too.

# Conclusion

## *That's almost it guys, but it's not the end.*

You've got the foundations you need, now it is time to build on them, using the knowledge you have. You now know what's going on with your hormones, the effect that midlife is potentially having on your mind, body and emotions, but you also have the tools required to optimise the symptoms and work in line with those hormonal changes.

The 30-day plan is but a mere introduction to what you can achieve with lifestyle factors to feel better in body and mind, but follow it, and you'll get results.

Commit to regular exercise and healthy balanced nutrition, keep checking on your goals and continue to set new ones. Make detailed plans to achieve them, and keep visualising your new future. Your goal is to step into the man you want to be, the man that you know you can be.

Use the principles and information to build out your routines and habits so you can embrace this part of your life with joy, energy and vigour.

Remember, life is also about having fun.

If you're inspired and want to know more, or you'd like a more in depth programme, or you're even considering one to one coaching with me, then just reach out.

# A Final Word

*There's a lot to take in here, I know that. Don't be overwhelmed. This book is designed to increase your knowledge and awareness around both your mind and body, to give you foundations you can build on.*

The more you can adhere to what's in here and the more closely you follow the programme, the better, but find what works for you and your life and goals.

I never want you to feel "not enough". Have self-compassion, make the choices that feel good for your long term aspirations and health and above all, be compassionate with yourself.

I have one last thing to ask, and that is to speak to other men about this stuff. Let's open the conversation. The more we can talk to each other and voice how we feel, the more supported we'll feel and the more our feelings will be normalised. No one should feel alone when it comes to managing midlife.

**Let's Stand Together.**

## Acknowledgments

Writing a book like this really is a team effort, so I'd like to thank the whole team at Synergy publishers, and in particular Suzi Wooldridge and Carolyn Andrews for their belief in the project. I'd like to thank the PR team at Read Maxwell for their work in getting the message out. Then there's my patient and fabulous editor Nicole Howes who helped craft the message in such a brilliant fashion - thank you. Last but definitely not least, a huge thank you to my wife Claire for her belief in me, in this book, for giving me the time and space to create it, and for being such an inspiring light to me and to so many others. Thank you. X

# Next Steps

There are plenty of free resources that accompany this book (workout videos, guided meditations, recipes and more), all designed to help you get the most from your journey.

You can grab them all here:
themidlifementors.com

Let's connect on social or in person:

**Podcast**
https://themidlifementors.com/podcast-2

**Linkedin**
https://www.linkedin.com/in/jamesdavis

**Instagram**
https://www.instagram.com/midlifementors

**Tik Tok**
https://www.tiktok.com/@themidlifementors

**Facebook**
https://www.facebook.com/themidlifementors

**Youtube**
https://www.youtube.com/c/themidlifementors

I will leave you with this final question,
**how do you want your tomorrow to look?**

# References

Age UK Loneliness Research and Resources. 2021.
https://www.ageuk.org.uk/our-impact/policy-research/loneliness-research-and-resources/

Albalooshi, S., Moeini-Jazani, M., Fennis, B. M., & Warlop, L. (2020). Reinstating the Resourceful Self: When and How Self-Affirmations Improve Executive Performance of the Powerless. Personality and Social Psychology Bulletin, 46(2), 189-203. https://doi.org/10.1177/0146167219853840.
https://journals.sagepub.com/doi/full/10.1177/0146167219853840

Ahmadizad S, Avansar AS, Ebrahim K, Avandi M, Ghasemikaram M. The effects of short-term high-intensity interval training vs. moderate-intensity continuous training on plasma levels of nesfatin-1 and inflammatory markers. Horm Mol Biol Clin Investig. 2015 Mar;21(3):165-73. doi: 10.1515/hmbci-2014-0038. PMID: 25581765.
https://pubmed.ncbi.nlm.nih.gov/25581765/

Akın S, Mucuk S, Öztürk A, Mazıcıoğlu M, Göçer Ş, Arguvanlı S, Şafak ED. Muscle function-dependent sarcopenia and cut-off values of possible predictors in community-dwelling Turkish elderly: calf circumference, midarm muscle circumference and walking speed. Eur J Clin Nutr. 2015 Oct;69(10):1087-90. doi: 10.1038/ejcn.2015.42. Epub 2015 Mar 18. PMID: 25782425. https://pubmed.ncbi.nlm.nih.gov/25782425/

Allen AP, Kennedy PJ, Cryan JF, Dinan TG, Clarke G. Biological and psychological markers of stress in humans: focus on the Trier Social Stress Test. Neurosci Biobehav Rev. 2014 Jan;38:94-124. doi: 10.1016/j.neubiorev.2013.11.005. Epub 2013 Nov 14. PMID: 24239854. https://pubmed.ncbi.nlm.nih.gov/24239854/

Almeida DM, Wethington E, Kessler RC. The daily inventory of stressful events: an interview-based approach for measuring daily stressors. Assessment. 2002 Mar;9(1):41-55. doi: 10.1177/1073191102091006. PMID: 11911234.
https://pubmed.ncbi.nlm.nih.gov/11911234/

Almeida, D. M., & Horn, M. C. (2004). Is Daily Life More Stressful during Middle Adulthood? In O. G. Brim, C. D. Ryff, & R. C. Kessler (Eds.), How healthy are we?: A national study of well-being at midlife (pp. 425–451). The University of Chicago Press. https://awspntest.apa.org/record/2004-00121-015

American Foundation for Suicide Prevention, Suicide Statistics. 2022. https://afsp.org/suicide-statistics/

Apoor S. Gami, Brandi J. Witt, Daniel E. Howard, Patricia J. Erwin, Lisa A. Gami, Virend K. Somers, Victor M. Montori, Metabolic Syndrome and Risk of Incident Cardiovascular Events and Death: A Systematic Review and Meta-Analysis of Longitudinal Studies, Journal of the American College of Cardiology, Volume 49, Issue 4, 2007, Pages 403-414, ISSN 0735-1097,

https://doi.org/10.1016/j.jacc.2006.09.032.
https://www.sciencedirect.com/science/article/pii/S0735109706026581

Armitage CJ, Harris PR, Hepton G, Napper L. Self-affirmation increases acceptance of health-risk information among UK adult smokers with low socioeconomic status. Psychol Addict Behav. 2008 Mar;22(1):88-95. doi: 10.1037/0893-164X.22.1.88. PMID: 18298234. https://pubmed.ncbi.nlm.nih.gov/18298234/

Arsalidou M, Pascual-Leone J, Johnson J, Morris D, Taylor MJ. A balancing act of the brain: activations and deactivations driven by cognitive load. Brain Behav. 2013 May;3(3):273-85. doi: 10.1002/brb3.128. Epub 2013 Apr 2. PMID: 23785659; PMCID: PMC3683287. https://pubmed.ncbi.nlm.nih.gov/23785659/

Aviva Newsroom As many as 16 million UK adults* are suffering from sleepless nights as a third (31%) say they have insomnia. 2017.
https://www.aviva.com/newsroom/news-releases/2017/10/Sleepless-cities-revealed-as-one-in-three-adults-suffer-from-insomnia/

Baltes PB, Baltes MM. Psychological perspectives on successful aging: The model of selective optimization with compensation. In: Baltes PB, Baltes MM, eds. Successful Aging: Perspectives from the Behavioral Sciences. European Network on Longitudinal Studies on Individual Development. Cambridge University Press; 1990:1-34. https://www.cambridge.org/core/books/abs/successful-aging/psychological-perspectives-on-successful-aging-the-model-of-selective-optimization-with-compensation/EAE9389C90617AE014260735DFFCEF82

Barrett-Connor E. The Rancho Bernardo Study: 40 years studying why women have less heart disease than men and how diabetes modifies women's usual cardiac protection. Glob Heart. 2013 Jun 1;8(2):10.1016/j.gheart.2012.12.002. doi: 10.1016/j.gheart.2012.12.002. PMID: 24187655; PMCID: PMC3810980.
https://www.ncbi.nlm.nih.gov/pmc/articles/PMC3810980/

Barry, J, Male mid-life crisis: causes, coping and meaning. The Centre For Male Psychology. 2023.
https://www.centreformalepsychology.com/male-psychology-magazine-listings/male-mid-life-crisis-causes-coping-and-meaning

BBC, How Pollution is Causing a Male Fertility Crisis. 2023.
https://www.bbc.com/future/article/20230327-how-pollution-is-causing-a-male-fertility-crisis

Bellavia A, Larsson SC, Bottai M, Wolk A, Orsini N. Fruit and vegetable consumption and all-cause mortality: a dose-response analysis. Am J Clin Nutr. 2013 Aug;98(2):454-9. doi: 10.3945/ajcn.112.056119. Epub 2013 Jun 26. PMID: 23803880. https://pubmed.ncbi.nlm.nih.gov/23803880/

Beutel, M. E., Glaesmer, H., Wiltink, J., Marian, H., & Brähler, E. (2009). Life satisfaction, anxiety, depression and resilience across the life span of men. The Aging Male, 13(1), 32–39. https://doi.org/10.3109/13685530903296698. https://www.tandfonline.com/doi/full/10.3109/13685530903296698

Bhasin S. Secular decline in male reproductive function: Is manliness threatened? J Clin Endocrinol Metab. 2007 Jan;92(1):44-5. doi: 10.1210/jc.2006-2438. PMID: 17209224. https://pubmed.ncbi.nlm.nih.gov/17209224/

Bikou A, Dermiki-Gkana F, Penteris M, Constantinides TK, Kontogiorgis C. A systematic review of the effect of semaglutide on lean mass: insights from clinical trials. Expert Opin Pharmacother. 2024 Apr;25(5):611-619. doi: 10.1080/14656566.2024.2343092. Epub 2024 Apr 18. PMID: 38629387.
https://pubmed.ncbi.nlm.nih.gov/38629387/

Blanchflower DG, Graham CL. The Mid-Life Dip in Well-Being: a Critique. Soc Indic Res. 2022;161(1):287-344. doi: 10.1007/s11205-021-02773-w. Epub 2021 Oct 19. PMID: 34690403; PMCID: PMC8525618.
https://www.ncbi.nlm.nih.gov/pmc/articles/PMC8525618/

Blanchflower DG, Oswald AJ. Is well-being U-shaped over the life cycle? Soc Sci Med. 2008 Apr;66(8):1733-49. doi: 10.1016/j.socscimed.2008.01.030. Epub 2008 Mar 7. PMID: 18316146.
https://pubmed.ncbi.nlm.nih.gov/18316146/

# REFERENCES

BodyScan, Body Fat Percentage: What is healthy? 2022. https://bodyscanuk.com/blog/body-fat-percentage-what-is-healthy/

Bouras, Andrew (2024) "Transcending Fear: The Power of Mindful Affirmations and Purposeful Action," Be Still: Vol. 8, Article 16. Available at: https://nsuworks.nova.edu/bestill/vol8/iss1/16

Boysen-Rotelli, Sheila & Cherry, M. & Amerie, W. & Takagawa, M.. (2018). Organisational coaching outcomes: A comparison of a practitioner survey and key findings from the literature. International Journal of Evidence Based Coaching and Mentoring. 16. 159-166. 10.24384/000475.

British Heart Foundation UK Factsheet 2024. https://www.bhf.org.uk/-/media/files/for-professionals/research/heart-statistics/bhf-cvd-statistics-uk-factsheet.pdf

Brott SRJ, Ng KL, Prostate Cancer, Chapter 1 The Epidemiology of Prostate Cancer, 2021. https://www.ncbi.nlm.nih.gov/books/NBK571326/

Camilleri GM, Méjean C, Bellisle F, Andreeva VA, Kesse-Guyot E, Hercberg S, Péneau S. Intuitive eating is inversely associated with body weight status in the general population-based NutriNet-Santé study. Obesity (Silver Spring). 2016 May;24(5):1154-61. doi: 10.1002/oby.21440. Epub 2016 Mar 17. PMID: 26991542. https://pubmed.ncbi.nlm.nih.gov/26991542/

Camilleri GM, Méjean C, Bellisle F, Andreeva VA, Kesse-Guyot E, Hercberg S, Péneau S. Intuitive eating is inversely associated with body weight status in the general population-based NutriNet-Santé study. Obesity (Silver Spring). 2016 May;24(5):1154-61. doi: 10.1002/oby.21440. Epub 2016 Mar 17. PMID: 26991542. https://pubmed.ncbi.nlm.nih.gov/26991542/

Cancer Research UK, Prostate Cancer Statistics 2024. https://www.cancerresearchuk.org/health-professional/cancer-statistics/statistics-by-cancer-type/prostate-cancer

Cancer Research UK 2024 https://www.cancerresearchuk.org/health-professional/cancer-statistics/statistics-by-cancer-type/prostate-cancer/incidence#heading-Zero

Chang M, Jonsson PV, Snaedal J, Bjornsson S, Saczynski JS, Aspelund T, Eiriksdottir G, Jonsdottir MK, Lopez OL, Harris TB, Gudnason V, Launer LJ. The effect of midlife physical activity on cognitive function among older adults: AGES--Reykjavik Study. J Gerontol A Biol Sci Med Sci. 2010 Dec;65(12):1369-74. doi: 10.1093/gerona/glq152. Epub 2010 Aug 30. PMID: 20805238; PMCID: PMC2990266. https://pubmed.ncbi.nlm.nih.gov/20805238/

Chronic stress puts your health at risk, Mayo Clinic, 2024. https://www.mayoclinic.org/healthy-lifestyle/stress-management/in-depth/stress/art-20046037

Chu B, Marwaha K, Sanvictores T, et al. Physiology, Stress Reaction. [Updated 2024 May 7]. In: StatPearls [Internet]. Treasure Island (FL): StatPearls Publishing; 2024 Jan-. Available from: https://www.ncbi.nlm.nih.gov/books/NBK541120/

Cipher, Workplace Stress Statistics in the UK in 2024. https://www.ciphr.com/infographics/workplace-stress-statistics

Cohen GL, Sherman DK. The psychology of change: self-affirmation and social psychological intervention. Annu Rev Psychol. 2014;65:333-71. doi: 10.1146/annurev-psych-010213-115137. PMID: 24405362. https://pubmed.ncbi.nlm.nih.gov/24405362/

Corfe, S. Sheperd, Social Market Foundation, Gendered Experiences Of Obesity. 2021. https://www.smf.co.uk/wp-content/uploads/2021/11/Gendered-experiences-of-obesity-Nov-2021.pdf

Craig BW, Brown R, Everhart J. Effects of progressive resistance training on growth hormone and testosterone levels in young and elderly subjects. Mech Ageing Dev. 1989 Aug;49(2):159-69. doi: 10.1016/0047-6374(89)90099-7. PMID: 2796409. https://pubmed.ncbi.nlm.nih.gov/2796409/

De Coninck S, Aben B, Van den Bussche E, Mariën P, Van Overwalle F. Embodying Stressful Events: No Difference in Subjective Arousal and Neural Correlates Related to Immersion, Interoception, and Embodied Mentalization. Front Behav Neurosci. 2021 May 13;15:640482. doi: 10.3389/fnbeh.2021.640482. PMID: 34054442; PMCID: PMC8161507. https://www.ncbi.nlm.nih.gov/pmc/articles/PMC8161507/

Department for Digital, Culture, Media & Sport, Wellbeing and Loneliness - Community Life Survey 2020/21. https://www.gov.uk/government/statistics/community-life-survey-202021-wellbeing-and-loneliness/wellbeing-and-loneliness-community-life-survey-202021

Diabetes.co.uk.Insulin Resistance. 2023. https://www.diabetes.co.uk/insulin-resistance.html

Ditzenberger GL, Lake JE, Kitch DW, Kantor A, Muthupillai R, Moser C, Belaunzaran-Zamudio PF, Brown TT, Corey K, Landay AL, Avihingsanon A, Sattler FR, Erlandson KM. Effects of Semaglutide on Muscle Structure and Function in the SLIM LIVER Study. Clin Infect Dis. 2024 Jul 24:ciae384. doi: 10.1093/cid/ciae384. Epub ahead of print. PMID: 39046173. https://pubmed.ncbi.nlm.nih.gov/39046173/

Drink Aware Alcohol Consumption UK. 2024. https://www.drinkaware.co.uk/research/alcohol-facts-and-data/alcohol-consumption-uk

Drink Aware, Alcohol and Stress, 2024. https://www.drinkaware.co.uk/facts/health-effects-of-alcohol/mental-health/alcohol-and-stress

Dr. Shilpa Raka, . (2023). NURTURING THE MIND: THE POWER OF POSITIVE AFFIRMATIONS IN ENHANCING PSYCHOLOGICAL WELL-BEING. American Journal of Philological Sciences, 3(05), 43–47. https://doi.org/10.37547/ajps/Volume03Issue05-08

Elderly have lower protein digestion and absorption? Nutrition Tactics. 2022. https://www.nutritiontactics.com/elderly-have-lower-protein-digestion-and-absorption/

Emily H. Feig, Christopher M. Celano, Christina N. Massey, Wei-Jean Chung, Perla Romero, Lauren E. Harnedy, Jeff C. Huffman, Association of Midlife Status With Response to a Positive Psychology Intervention in Patients With Acute Coronary Syndrome, Journal of the Academy of Consultation-Liaison Psychiatry, Volume 62, Issue 2, 2021, Pages 220-227, ISSN 2667-2960. https://doi.org/10.1016/j.psym.2020.06.002. https://www.sciencedirect.com/science/article/pii/S0033318220301882

Fain E, Weatherford C. Comparative study of millennials' (age 20-34 years) grip and lateral pinch with the norms. J Hand Ther. 2016 Oct-Dec;29(4):483-488. doi: 10.1016/j.jht.2015.12.006. Epub 2016 Jan 11. Erratum in: J Hand Ther. 2020 Jan - Mar;33(1):150. doi: 10.1016/j.jht.2020.03.006. PMID: 26869476. https://pubmed.ncbi.nlm.nih.gov/26869476/

Falcone PH, Tai CY, Carson LR, Joy JM, Mosman MM, McCann TR, Crona KP, Kim MP, Moon JR. Caloric expenditure of aerobic, resistance, or combined high-intensity interval training using a hydraulic resistance system in healthy men. J Strength Cond Res. 2015 Mar;29(3):779-85. doi: 10.1519/JSC.0000000000000661. PMID: 25162652. https://pubmed.ncbi.nlm.nih.gov/25162652/

Fetissov SO. Role of the gut microbiota in host appetite control: bacterial growth to animal feeding behaviour. Nat Rev Endocrinol. 2017 Jan;13(1):11-25. doi: 10.1038/nrendo.2016.150. Epub 2016 Sep 12. PMID: 27616451. https://pubmed.ncbi.nlm.nih.gov/27616451/

Finlay-Jones R, Brown GW. types of stressful life event and the onset of anxiety and depressive disorders. Psychol Med. 1981 Nov;11(4):803-15. doi: 10.1017/s0033291700041301. PMID: 7323236. https://pubmed.ncbi.nlm.nih.gov/7323236/

Foscolou A, D'Cunha NM, Naumovski N, Tyrovolas S, Chrysohoou C, Rallidis L, Matalas AL, Sidossis LS, Panagiotakos D. The Association between Whole Grain Products Consumption and Successful Aging: A Combined Analysis of MEDIS and ATTICA Epidemiological Studies. Nutrients. 2019 May 29;11(6):1221. doi: 10.3390/nu11061221. PMID: 31146435; PMCID: PMC6627753. https://www.ncbi.nlm.nih.gov/pmc/articles/PMC6627753/

Freund AM, Ritter JO. Midlife crisis: a debate. Gerontology. 2009;55(5):582-91. doi: 10.1159/000227322. Epub 2009 Jul 2. PMID: 19571526. https://pubmed.ncbi.nlm.nih.gov/19571526/

FSHD Society 2024. https://www.fshdsociety.org/2024/08/12/muscle-loss-with-ozempic-and-similar-drugs/

Fui MN, Dupuis P, Grossmann M. Lowered testosterone in male obesity: mechanisms, morbidity and management. Asian J Androl. 2014 Mar-Apr;16(2):223-31. doi: 10.4103/1008-682X.122365. PMID: 24407187; PMCID: PMC3955331. https://www.ncbi.nlm.nih.gov/pmc/articles/PMC3955331/

Gallup, U.S. Depression Rates Reach New Highs, 2017.
https://news.gallup.com/poll/505745/depression-rates-reach-new-highs.aspx

Gambler, V, Chad, N. K. Psychological experiences of midlife, Indian Journal Of Positive Psychology, Vol 4, Iss 1, 26-31, 2013.
https://www.proquest.com/openview/225a7c8272b90136bbec26f774568008/1?pq-origsite=gscholar&cbl=2032133

Glenn R. Cunningham, Alvin M. Matsumoto, Ronald Swerdloff, Low Testosterone and Men's Health, The Journal of Clinical Endocrinology & Metabolism, Volume 89, Issue 5, 1 May 2004, Page E2, https://doi.org/10.1210/jcem.89.5.9997

Glycanage, Biological Age: The Ultimate Guide. 2024. https://glycanage.com/self-care/lifestyle/biological-age

Godoy LD, Rossignoli MT, Delfino-Pereira P, Garcia-Cairasco N, de Lima Umeoka EH. A Comprehensive Overview on Stress Neurobiology: Basic Concepts and Clinical Implications. Front Behav Neurosci. 2018 Jul 3;12:127. doi: 10.3389/fnbeh.2018.00127. PMID: 30034327; PMCID: PMC6043787. https://pubmed.ncbi.nlm.nih.gov/30034327/

Goodale T, Sadhu A, Petak S, Robbins R. Testosterone and the Heart. Methodist Debakey Cardiovasc J. 2017 Apr-Jun;13(2):68-72. doi: 10.14797/mdcj-13-2-68. PMID: 28740585; PMCID: PMC5512682. https://www.ncbi.nlm.nih.gov/pmc/articles/PMC5512682/

Gordon, I. J. (1972). Success and Accountability. Childhood Education, 48(7), 338–347. https://doi.org/10.1080/00094056.1972.10727393. https://www.tandfonline.com/doi/pdf/10.1080/00094056.1972.10727393

Gorissen SHM, Trommelen J, Kouw IWK, Holwerda AM, Pennings B, Groen BBL, Wall BT, Churchward-Venne TA, Horstman AMH, Koopman R, Burd NA, Fuchs CJ, Dirks ML, Res PT, Senden JMG, Steijns JMJM, de Groot LCPGM, Verdijk LB, van Loon LJC. Protein Type, Protein Dose, and Age Modulate Dietary Protein Digestion and Phenylalanine Absorption Kinetics and Plasma Phenylalanine Availability in Humans. J Nutr. 2020 Aug 1;150(8):2041-2050. doi: 10.1093/jn/nxaa024. PMID: 32069356; PMCID: PMC7398787. https://pubmed.ncbi.nlm.nih.gov/32069356/

Grzywacz JG. Work-family spillover and health during midlife: is managing conflict everything? Am J Health Promot. 2000 Mar-Apr;14(4):236-43. doi: 10.4278/0890-1171-14.4.236. PMID: 10915535. https://pubmed.ncbi.nlm.nih.gov/10915535/

Hackney AC. Hypogonadism in Exercising Males: Dysfunction or Adaptive-Regulatory Adjustment? Front Endocrinol (Lausanne). 2020 Jan 31;11:11. doi: 10.3389/fendo.2020.00011. PMID: 32082255; PMCID: PMC7005256. https://pubmed.ncbi.nlm.nih.gov/32082255/

Hall KD, Ayuketah A, Brychta R, Cai H, Cassimatis T, Chen KY, Chung ST, Costa E, Courville A, Darcey V, Fletcher LA, Forde CG, Gharib AM, Guo J, Howard R, Joseph PV, McGehee S, Ouwerkerk R, Raisinger K, Rozga I, Stagliano M, Walter M, Walter PJ, Yang S, Zhou M. Ultra-Processed Diets Cause Excess Calorie Intake and Weight Gain: An Inpatient Randomized Controlled Trial of Ad Libitum Food Intake. Cell Metab. 2019 Jul 2;30(1):67-77.e3. doi: 10.1016/j.cmet.2019.05.008. Epub 2019 May 16. Erratum in: Cell Metab. 2019 Jul 2;30(1):226. doi: 10.1016/j.cmet.2019.05.020. Erratum in: Cell Metab. 2020 Oct 6;32(4):690. doi: 10.1016/j.cmet.2020.08.014. PMID: 31105044; PMCID: PMC7946062. https://pubmed.ncbi.nlm.nih.gov/31105044/

Hayes LD, Herbert P, Sculthorpe NF, Grace FM. Exercise training improves free testosterone in lifelong sedentary aging men. Endocr Connect. 2017 Jul;6(5):306-310. doi: 10.1530/EC-17-0082. Epub 2017 May 17. PMID: 28515052; PMCID: PMC5510446. https://www.ncbi.nlm.nih.gov/pmc/articles/PMC5510446/

He J, Wang S, Zhou M, Yu W, Zhang Y, He X. Phytoestrogens and risk of prostate cancer: a meta-analysis of observational studies. World J Surg Oncol. 2015 Jul 31;13:231. doi: 10.1186/s12957-015-0648-9. PMID: 26228387; PMCID: PMC4521376. https://www.ncbi.nlm.nih.gov/pmc/articles/PMC4521376/#:~:text=Conclusions,especially%20genistein%20and%20daidzein%20intake

Health And Safety Executive, LFS - Labour Force Survey - Self-Reported Work-Related Ill Health and Workplace Injuries: Index of LFS Tables. 2023 https://www.hse.gov.uk/Statistics/lfs/index.htm

Health And Safety Executive, Work-related Ill Health and Occupational Disease in Great Britain. 2024. https://www.hse.gov.uk/statistics/causdis/index.htm

Healthline, 10 Ways to Boost Human Growth Hormone (HGH) Naturally. 2023. https://www.healthline.com/nutrition/11-ways-to-increase-hgh

Healthline, Does Working Out Increase Testosterone Levels? 2022. https://www.healthline.com/health/does-working-out-increase-testosterone

Healthline, Leptin and Leptin Resistance: Everything You Need to Know. 2023. https://www.healthline.com/nutrition/leptin-101

Healthline 2024: https://www.healthline.com/health-news/ozempic-muscle-mass-loss

Hirotsu C, Tufik S, Andersen ML. Interactions between sleep, stress, and metabolism: From physiological to pathological conditions. Sleep Sci. 2015 Nov;8(3):143-52. doi: 10.1016/j.slsci.2015.09.002. Epub 2015 Sep 28. PMID: 26779321; PMCID: PMC4688585. https://www.ncbi.nlm.nih.gov/pmc/articles/PMC4688585/

# REFERENCES

Huffman JC, Beale EE, Celano CM, Beach SR, Belcher AM, Moore SV, Suarez L, Motiwala SR, Gandhi PU, Gaggin HK, Januzzi JL. Effects of Optimism and Gratitude on Physical Activity, Biomarkers, and Readmissions After an Acute Coronary Syndrome: The Gratitude Research in Acute Coronary Events Study. Circ Cardiovasc Qual Outcomes. 2016 Jan;9(1):55-63. doi: 10.1161/CIRCOUTCOMES.115.002184. Epub 2015 Dec 8. PMID: 26646818; PMCID: PMC4720551. https://www.ncbi.nlm.nih.gov/pmc/articles/PMC4720551/

International Osteoporosis Foundation, SCORECARD FOR OSTEOPOROSIS IN EUROPE (SCOPE) Epidemiology, Burden, and Treatment of Osteoporosis in the United Kingdom. 2021. https://www.osteoporosis.foundation/sites/iofbonehealth/files/scope-2021/UK%20report.pdf

ISSN 0735-1097. https://www.sciencedirect.com/science/article/pii/S0735109706026581

Jelleyman C, Yates T, O'Donovan G, Gray LJ, King JA, Khunti K, Davies MJ. The effects of high-intensity interval training on glucose regulation and insulin resistance: a meta-analysis. Obes Rev. 2015 Nov;16(11):942-61. doi: 10.1111/obr.12317. PMID: 26481101. https://pubmed.ncbi.nlm.nih.gov/26481101/

Jeng HA. Exposure to endocrine disrupting chemicals and male reproductive health. Front Public Health. 2014 Jun 5;2:55. doi: 10.3389/fpubh.2014.00055. PMID: 24926476; PMCID: PMC4046332. https://www.ncbi.nlm.nih.gov/pmc/articles/PMC4046332/

Jiannine LM. An investigation of the relationship between physical fitness, self-concept, and sexual functioning. J Educ Health Promot. 2018 May 3;7:57. doi: 10.4103/jehp.jehp_157_17. PMID: 29922686; PMCID: PMC5963213. https://www.ncbi.nlm.nih.gov/pmc/articles/PMC5963213/

Joëls M, Baram TZ. The neuro-symphony of stress. Nat Rev Neurosci. 2009 Jun;10(6):459-66. doi: 10.1038/nrn2632. PMID: 19339973; PMCID: PMC2844123. https://pubmed.ncbi.nlm.nih.gov/19339973/

Julie L. Ji, Stephanie Burnett Heyes, Colin MacLeod, Emily A. Holmes,

Emotional Mental Imagery as Simulation of Reality: Fear and Beyond—A Tribute to Peter Lang, Behavior Therapy, Volume 47, Issue 5, 2016, Pages 702-719, ISSN 0005-7894,

https://doi.org/10.1016/j.beth.2015.11.004. https://www.sciencedirect.com/science/article/pii/S0005789415001239

Kahneman, D, The Lancet, Wellbeing: an idea whose time has come, Volume 366, Issue 9495p1412October 22, 2005. https://www.thelancet.com/journals/lancet/article/PIIS0140-6736(05)67578-2/fulltext

Kim, S. Y., Fouad, N., Maeda, H., Xie, H., & Nazan, N. (2018). Midlife Work and Psychological Well-Being: A Test of the Psychology of Working Theory. Journal of Career Assessment, 26(3), 413-424. https://doi.org/10.1177/1069072717714538. https://journals.sagepub.com/doi/abs/10.1177/1069072717714538

Kivimäki, M., Kawachi, I. Work Stress as a Risk Factor for Cardiovascular Disease. Curr Cardiol Rep 17, 74 (2015). https://doi.org/10.1007/s11886-015-0630-8

Knudsen LB, Lau J. The Discovery and Development of Liraglutide and Semaglutide. Front Endocrinol (Lausanne). 2019 Apr 12;10:155. doi: 10.3389/fendo.2019.00155. PMID: 31031702; PMCID: PMC6474072. https://pubmed.ncbi.nlm.nih.gov/31031702/

Kriakous SA, Elliott KA, Lamers C, Owen R. The Effectiveness of Mindfulness-Based Stress Reduction on the Psychological Functioning of Healthcare Professionals: a Systematic Review. Mindfulness (N Y). 2021;12(1):1-28. doi: 10.1007/s12671-020-01500-9. Epub 2020 Sep 24. PMID: 32989406; PMCID: PMC7511255. https://www.ncbi.nlm.nih.gov/pmc/articles/PMC7511255/

Lacey, J.I., Appley, M.H. and Trumbull, R., 1967. Psychological stress.

Lachman ME, Teshale S, Agrigoroaei S. Midlife as a Pivotal Period in the Life Course: Balancing Growth and Decline at the Crossroads of Youth and Old Age. Int J Behav Dev. 2015 Jan 1;39(1):20-31. doi: 10.1177/0165025414533223. PMID: 25580043; PMCID: PMC4286887. https://www.ncbi.nlm.nih.gov/pmc/articles/PMC4286887/

Lachman, M. E. Handbook of Midlife Development, Wiley, 2001. https://www.brandeis.edu/psychology/lachman/pdfs/handbkofmidlifedevel.pdf

Leproult R, Copinschi G, Buxton O, Van Cauter E. Sleep loss results in an elevation of cortisol levels the next evening. Sleep. 1997 Oct;20(10):865-70. PMID: 9415946. https://pubmed.ncbi.nlm.nih.gov/9415946/

Leproult R, Van Cauter E. Effect of 1 week of sleep restriction on testosterone levels in young healthy men. JAMA. 2011 Jun 1;305(21):2173-4. doi: 10.1001/jama.2011.710. PMID: 21632481; PMCID: PMC4445839. https://www.ncbi.nlm.nih.gov/pmc/articles/PMC4445839/

Liddon, L., & Barry, J. (2021). Perspectives in male psychology: An introduction. John Wiley & Sons. ISBN: 978-1-119-68535-7. https://www.wiley.com/en-gb/Perspectives+in+Male+Psychology%3A+An+Introduction-p-9781119685357

Lohman T, Bains G, Cole S, Gharibvand L, Berk L, Lohman E. High-Intensity interval training reduces transcriptomic age: A randomized controlled trial. Aging Cell. 2023 Jun;22(6):e13841. doi: 10.1111/acel.13841. Epub 2023 Apr 20. PMID: 37078430; PMCID: PMC10265161. https://www.ncbi.nlm.nih.gov/pmc/articles/PMC10265161/

Lokeshwar SD, Patel P, Fantus RJ, Halpern J, Chang C, Kargi AY, Ramasamy R. Decline in Serum Testosterone Levels Among Adolescent and Young Adult Men in the USA. Eur Urol Focus. 2021 Jul;7(4):886-889. doi: 10.1016/j.euf.2020.02.006. Epub 2020 Feb 18. PMID: 32081788. https://pubmed.ncbi.nlm.nih.gov/32081788/

Lyubomirsky S, King L, Diener E. The benefits of frequent positive affect: does happiness lead to success? Psychol Bull. 2005 Nov;131(6):803-55. doi: 10.1037/0033-2909.131.6.803. PMID: 16351326. https://pubmed.ncbi.nlm.nih.gov/16351326/

Mann U, Shiff B, Patel P. Reasons for worldwide decline in male fertility. Curr Opin Urol. 2020 May;30(3):296-301. doi: 10.1097/MOU.0000000000000745. PMID: 32168194. https://pubmed.ncbi.nlm.nih.gov/32168194/

McKeown NM, Meigs JB, Liu S, Wilson PW, Jacques PF. Whole-grain intake is favorably associated with metabolic risk factors for type 2 diabetes and cardiovascular disease in the Framingham Offspring Study. Am J Clin Nutr. 2002 Aug;76(2):390-8. doi: 10.1093/ajcn/76.2.390. PMID: 12145012. https://pubmed.ncbi.nlm.nih.gov/12145012/

McManus S, Bebbington P, Jenkins R, Brugha T. (eds.) (2016) Mental health and wellbeing in England: Adult Psychiatric Morbidity Survey 2014. Leeds: NHS Digital http://content.digital.nhs.uk/catalogue/PUB21748/apms-2014-full-rpt.pdf

MCQueen, A., & Klein, W. M. P. (2006). Experimental manipulations of self-affirmation: A systematic review. Self and Identity, 5(4), 289–354. https://doi.org/10.1080/15298860600805325. https://www.tandfonline.com/doi/abs/10.1080/15298860600805325

Medichecks, Why do Gen Z and millennial men have lower testosterone levels? 2024. https://www.medichecks.com/blogs/testosterone/why-do-gen-z-and-millennial-men-have-lower-testosterone

# REFERENCES

Mellor, D., Connaughton, C., McCabe, M. P., & Tatangelo, G. (2017). Better with age: A health promotion program for men at midlife. Psychology of Men & Masculinity, 18(1), 40–49.
https://doi.org/10.1037/men0000037 https://psycnet.apa.org/record/2016-07851-001

Men's Health Forum Annual Report 2017. https://www.menshealthforum.org.uk/annual-report-2017

Men's Health Forum Key Data Mental Health 2017. https://www.menshealthforum.org.uk/key-data-mental-health

Mental Health Foundation Stigma and discrimination. 2024.
https://www.mentalhealth.org.uk/explore-mental-health/a-z-topics/stigma-and-discrimination

Mental Health Foundation, Anxiety: Statistics. 2024.
https://www.mentalhealth.org.uk/explore-mental-health/statistics/anxiety-statistics

Mental Health Foundation, Stress: Statistics. 2019.
https://www.mentalhealth.org.uk/explore-mental-health/statistics/stress-statistics

Merrill, C. Andersen PhD, Executive Briefing: Case Study on the Return on Investment of Executive Coaching, MetrixGlobal, Nov 2001. https://www.slideshare.net/Dokkan/metrix-global-coaching-roi-briefing

MHFA England Mental Health Statistics 2020.
https://mhfaengland.org/mhfa-centre/research-and-evaluation/mental-health-statistics/

Mind Get It Off Your Chest Report 2019. https://www.mind.org.uk/media/6771/get-it-off-your-chest_a4_final.pdf

MInguez-Alarcón L, Chavarro JE, Mendiola J, Roca M, Tanrikut C, Vioque J, Jørgensen N, Torres-Cantero AM. Fatty acid intake in relation to reproductive hormones and testicular volume among young healthy men. Asian J Androl. 2017 Mar-Apr;19(2):184-190. doi: 10.4103/1008-682X.190323. PMID: 27834316; PMCID: PMC5312216.
https://www.ncbi.nlm.nih.gov/pmc/articles/PMC5312216/

Molly M. Shores, MD; Victoria M. Moceri, PhD; Kevin L. Sloan, MD; Alvin M. Matsumoto, MD; and Daniel R. Kivlahan, PhD, Low Testosterone Levels Predict Incident Depressive Illness in Older Men: Effects of Age and Medical Morbidity. The Journal Of Clinical Psychiatry. January 2005.
https://www.psychiatrist.com/jcp/low-testosterone-levels-predict-incident-depressive/

Morisano, Dominique,Hirsh, Jacob B.,Peterson, Jordan B.,Pihl, Robert O.,Shore, Bruce M.

Setting, elaborating, and reflecting on personal goals improves academic performance. Journal of Applied Psychology, Vol 95(2), Mar 2010, 255-264

Mund M, Mitte K. The costs of repression: a meta-analysis on the relation between repressive coping and somatic diseases. Health Psychol. 2012 Sep;31(5):640-9. doi: 10.1037/a0026257. Epub 2011 Nov 14. PMID: 22081940.
https://pubmed.ncbi.nlm.nih.gov/22081940/

Nakamura, J., Warren, M., Branand, B., Liu, PJ., Wheeler, B., Chan, T. (2014). Positive Psychology Across the Lifespan. In: Teramoto Pedrotti, J., Edwards, L. (eds) Perspectives on the Intersection of Multiculturalism and Positive Psychology. Cross-Cultural Advancements in Positive Psychology, vol 7. Springer, Dordrecht.
https://doi.org/10.1007/978-94-017-8654-6_8. https://link.springer.com/chapter/10.1007/978-94-017-8654-6_8

National Alliance On Mental Illness. Risk Of Suicide. 2021.
https://www.nami.org/About-Mental-Illness/Common-with-Mental-Illness/Risk-of-Suicide

National Institute Of Environmental Health Sciences. Endocrine Disruptors. 2024.
https://www.niehs.nih.gov/health/topics/agents/endocrine/index.cfm

Neeland IJ, Linge J, Birkenfeld AL. Changes in lean body mass with glucagon-like peptide-1-based therapies and mitigation strategies. Diabetes Obes Metab. 2024; 26(Suppl. 4): 16-27. doi:10.1111/dom.15728.
https://dom-pubs.onlinelibrary.wiley.com/doi/10.1111/dom.15728?af=R

Nelson CM, Bunge RG. Semen analysis: evidence for changing parameters of male fertility potential. Fertil Steril. 1974 Jun;25(6):503-7. doi: 10.1016/s0015-0282(16)40454-1. PMID: 4835605.
https://pubmed.ncbi.nlm.nih.gov/4835605/

NHS Cardiovascular Disease. 2024.
https://www.nhs.uk/conditions/cardiovascular-disease/#:~:text=age%20%E2%80%93%20CVD%20is%20most%20common,cholesterol%20and%20high%20blood%20pressure

NHS Digital Adult Psychiatric Morbidity Survey: Survey of Mental Health and Wellbeing, England, 2014.
https://webarchive.nationalarchives.gov.uk/ukgwa/20180328140249/http:/digital.nhs.uk/catalogue/PUB21748

NHS Digital Health Survey England Additional Analyses, Ethnicity and Health, 2011-2019 Experimental statistics, Fruit and Vegetable Consumption.
https://digital.nhs.uk/data-and-information/publications/statistical/health-survey-england-additional-analyses/ethnicity-and-health-2011-2019-experimental-statistics/fruit-and-vegetable-consumption

NHS Digital Health Survey for England, 2022 Part 1.
https://digital.nhs.uk/data-and-information/publications/statistical/health-survey-for-england/2022-part-1/adult-drinking

NHS Digital Mental Health Act Statistics Annual Figures. 2020.
https://files.digital.nhs.uk/99/3916C8/ment-heal-act-stat-eng-2019-20-summ-rep%20v1.1.pdf

NHS Digital, Health Survey for England, 2022 Part 2.
https://digital.nhs.uk/data-and-information/publications/statistical/health-survey-for-england/2022-part-2

NHS Metabolic Syndrome. 2024. https://www.nhs.uk/conditions/metabolic-syndrome/

NHS 2024 https://www.nhs.uk/conditions/prostate-cancer/symptoms/

Niehuas, L, University of South Africa. From crisis to awakening: an exploration of midlife experiences from a positive psychology perspective. 2019. https://core.ac.uk/download/pdf/219609628.pdf

Noetel M, Sanders T, Gallardo-GÃ³mez D, Taylor P, del Pozo Cruz B, van den Hoek D et al. Effect of exercise for depression: systematic review and network meta-analysis of randomised controlled trials BMJ 2024; 384 :e075847 doi:10.1136/bmj-2023-075847. https://www.bmj.com/content/384/bmj-2023-075847

Nuffield Trust Obesity 2023.
https://www.nuffieldtrust.org.uk/resource/obesity?gad_source=1&gclid=Cj0KCQjwpP63BhDYARIsAOQkATYR12JqfcxwFH2Zduzt8AzXJcn7fqjyTblaEpjBSWtiZ_jQyiNLYo8aAsO7EALw_wcB

Nyante SJ, Graubard BI, Li Y, McQuillan GM, Platz EA, Rohrmann S, Bradwin G, McGlynn KA. Trends in sex hormone concentrations in US males: 1988-1991 to 1999-2004. Int J Androl. 2012 Jun;35(3):456-66. doi: 10.1111/j.1365-2605.2011.01230.x. Epub 2011 Dec 13. PMID: 22150314; PMCID: PMC4137971.
https://pubmed.ncbi.nlm.nih.gov/22150314/

# REFERENCES

ONS 2017.Personal well-being in the UK.
https://www.ons.gov.uk/peoplepopulationandcommunity/wellbeing/bulletins/measuringnationalwellbeing/october2016toseptember2017

ONS 2019. Suicides in the UK: 2018 registrations.
https://www.ons.gov.uk/peoplepopulationandcommunity/birthsdeathsandmarriages/deaths/bulletins/suicidesintheunitedkingdom/2018registrations

ONS 2020. Suicides in England and Wales. 2019 registrations.
https://www.ons.gov.uk/peoplepopulationandcommunity/birthsdeathsandmarriages/deaths/bulletins/suicidesintheunitedkingdom/2019registrations

ONS Cenus 2021.
https://www.ons.gov.uk/peoplepopulationandcommunity/birthsdeathsandmarriages/deaths/bulletins/suicidesintheunitedkingdom/2021registrations

ONS Deaths registered in England and Wales 2021.
https://www.ons.gov.uk/peoplepopulationandcommunity/birthsdeathsandmarriages/deaths/bulletins/deathsregistrationsummarytables/2022

ONS Ischaemic heart diseases deaths including comorbidities, England and Wales: 2019 registrations (2019).
https://www.ons.gov.uk/peoplepopulationandcommunity/birthsdeathsandmarriages/deaths/bulletins/ischaemicheartdiseasesdeathsincludingcomorbiditiesenglandandwales/2019registrations

ONS Overview of violent crime and sexual offences 2021.
https://www.ons.gov.uk/peoplepopulationandcommunity/crimeandjustice/compendium/focusonviolentcrimeandsexualoffences/yearendingmarch2015/chapter1overviewofviolentcrimeandsexualoffences#characteristics-associated-with-being-a-victim

ONS Sickness absence in the UK labour market: February 2014.
https://www.ons.gov.uk/employmentandlabourmarket/peopleinwork/labourproductivity/articles/sicknessabsenceinthelabourmarket/2014-02-25

Parsons, M. University Of Southern California .Positive Psychology Coaching and its Impact on Midlife Executives. 2016.
https://www.proquest.com/openview/c2e1f128a71bc96b98897ea01f211006/1?pq-origsite=gscholar&cbl=18750

Pascoe MC, Thompson DR, Jenkins ZM, Ski CF. Mindfulness mediates the physiological markers of stress: Systematic review and meta-analysis. J Psychiatr Res. 2017 Dec;95:156-178. doi: 10.1016/j.jpsychires.2017.08.004. Epub 2017 Aug 23. PMID: 28863392. https://pubmed.ncbi.nlm.nih.gov/28863392/

Pennings B, Groen B, de Lange A, Gijsen AP, Zorenc AH, Senden JM, van Loon LJ. Amino acid absorption and subsequent muscle protein accretion following graded intakes of whey protein in elderly men. Am J Physiol Endocrinol Metab. 2012 Apr 15;302(8):E992-9. doi: 10.1152/ajpendo.00517.2011. Epub 2012 Feb 14. PMID: 22338070.
https://pubmed.ncbi.nlm.nih.gov/22338070/

Phillips, J.J., & Phillips, P.P. ( 2007). Show me the money: The use of ROI in performance improvement, part 1. Performance Improvement, 46(9), 8–22. [DOI: 10.1002/pfi.160.] https://onlinelibrary.wiley.com/doi/10.1002/pfi.160

Plamen D. Penev, Association Between Sleep and Morning Testosterone Levels In Older Men, Sleep, Volume 30, Issue 4, April 2007, Pages 427–432.
https://academic.oup.com/sleep/article-abstract/30/4/427/2708195?redirectedFrom=fulltext

Pontzer H, Yamada Y, Sagayama H, Ainslie PN, Andersen LF, Anderson LJ, Arab L, Baddou I, Bedu-Addo K, Blaak EE, Blanc S, Bonomi AG, Bouten CVC, Bovet P, Buchowski MS, Butte NF, Camps SG, Close GL, Cooper JA, Cooper R, Das SK, Dugas LR, Ekelund U, Entringer S, Forrester T, Fudge BW, Goris AH, Gurven M, Hambly C, El Hamdouchi A, Hoos MB, Hu S, Joonas N, Joosen AM, Katzmarzyk P, Kempen KP, Kimura M, Kraus WE, Kushner RF, Lambert EV, Leonard WR, Lessan N, Martin C, Medin AC, Meijer EP, Morehen JC, Morton JP, Neuhouser ML, Nicklas TA, Ojiambo RM, Pietiläinen KH, Pitsiladis YP, Plange-Rhule J, Plasqui G, Prentice RL, Rabinovich RA, Racette SB, Raichlen DA, Ravussin E, Reynolds RM, Roberts SB, Schuit AJ, Sjödin AM, Stice E, Urlacher SS, Valenti G, Van Etten LM, Van Mil EA, Wells JCK, Wilson G, Wood BM, Yanovski J, Yoshida T, Zhang X, Murphy-Alford AJ, Loechl C, Luke AH, Rood J, Schoeller DA, Westerterp KR, Wong WW, Speakman JR; IAEA DLW Database Consortium. Daily energy expenditure through the human life course. Science. 2021 Aug 13;373(6556):808-812. doi: 10.1126/science.abe5017. PMID: 34385400; PMCID: PMC8370708. https://pubmed.ncbi.nlm.nih.gov/34385400/

Priory Group Men's mental health: 40% of men won't talk to anyone about their mental health. 2022. https://www.priorygroup.com/blog/40-of-men-wont-talk-to-anyone-about-their-mental-health

Public Health Collaboration. Dr David Unwin's Sugar Infographics. 2024. https://phcuk.org/sugar/

Rafael de Cabo, Ph.D., and Mark P. Mattson, Ph.D. New England Journal of Medicine, Volume 381 • Number 26 • December 26, 2019. Pages: 2541-2551. https://www.nejm.org/doi/full/10.1056/nejmra1905136

Prostate Cancer UK 2024. https://prostatecanceruk.org/prostate-information-and-support/risk-and-symptoms/about-prostate-cancer

Rauch, Jonathan, The Happiness Curve: Why Life Gets Better After 50, Bloomsbury, 2019.

Robert M Edinburgh, Helen E Bradley, Nurul-Fadhilah Abdullah, Scott L Robinson, Oliver J Chrzanowski-Smith, Jean-Philippe Walhin, Sophie Joanisse, Konstantinos N Manolopoulos, Andrew Philp, Aaron Hengist, Adrian Chabowski, Frances M Brodsky, Francoise Koumanov, James A Betts, Dylan Thompson, Gareth A Wallis, Javier T Gonzalez, Lipid Metabolism Links Nutrient-Exercise Timing to Insulin Sensitivity in Men Classified as Overweight or Obese, The Journal of Clinical Endocrinology & Metabolism, Volume 105, Issue 3, March 2020, Pages 660–676, https://doi.org/10.1210/clinem/dgz104

Roland, B. C., & Morris, J. L. (1986). Proposed Relation of Testosterone Levels to Male Suicides and Sudden Deaths. Psychological Reports, 59(1), 100-102. https://doi.org/10.2466/pr0.1986.59.1.100. https://journals.sagepub.com/doi/10.2466/pr0.1986.59.1.100

Sabag A, Najafi A, Michael S, Esgin T, Halaki M, Hackett D. The compatibility of concurrent high intensity interval training and resistance training for muscular strength and hypertrophy: a systematic review and meta-analysis. J Sports Sci. 2018 Nov;36(21):2472-2483. doi: 10.1080/02640414.2018.1464636. Epub 2018 Apr 16. PMID: 29658408. https://www.ncbi.nlm.nih.gov/pubmed/29658408

Samia Ahmed, Fatma Moussa, Akmal Moustafa, Doaa R. Ayoub, The Egyptian Journal of Neurology, Psychiatry and Neurosurgery, 2016. https://applications.emro.who.int/imemrf/105/Egypt-J-Neurol-Psychiatry-Neurosurg-2016-53-4-193-197-eng.pdf

Satizabal CL, Himali JJ, Beiser AS, Ramachandran V, Melo van Lent D, Himali D, Aparicio HJ, Maillard P, DeCarli CS, Harris WS, Seshadri S. Association of Red Blood Cell Omega-3 Fatty Acids With MRI Markers and Cognitive Function in Midlife: The Framingham Heart Study. Neurology. 2022 Dec 5;99(23):e2572-e2582. doi: 10.1212/WNL.0000000000201296. PMID: 36198518; PMCID: PMC9754651. https://www.neurology.org/doi/10.1212/WNL.0000000000201296

# REFERENCES

Satyjeet F, Naz S, Kumar V, Aung NH, Bansari K, Irfan S, Rizwan A. Psychological Stress as a Risk Factor for Cardiovascular Disease: A Case-Control Study. Cureus. 2020 Oct 1;12(10):e10757. doi: 10.7759/cureus.10757. PMID: 33150108; PMCID: PMC7603890. https://www.ncbi.nlm.nih.gov/pmc/articles/PMC7603890/

Schneiderman N, Ironson G, Siegel SD. Stress and health: psychological, behavioral, and biological determinants. Annu Rev Clin Psychol. 2005;1:607-28. doi: 10.1146/annurev.clinpsy.1.102803.144141. PMID: 17716101; PMCID: PMC2568977. https://www.ncbi.nlm.nih.gov/pmc/articles/PMC2568977/

Sherman, DK (Sherman, David K.) ; Cohen, GL (Cohen, Geoffrey L.) The psychology of self-defense: Self-affirmation theory. Advances in Experimental Social Psychology, Volume 38, Page 183 - 242. DOI: 10.1016/S0065-2601(06)38004-5

Schubert MM, Palumbo E, Seay RF, Spain KK, Clarke HE (2017) Energy compensation after sprint- and high-intensity interval training. PLoS ONE 12(12): e0189590. https://doi.org/10.1371/journal.pone.0189590. https://journals.plos.org/plosone/article?id=10.1371/journal.pone.0189590

Scientific American, Sperm Count Dropping in Western World, 2017. https://www.scientificamerican.com/article/sperm-count-dropping-in-western-world/

Seidler ZE, Rice SM, Ogrodniczuk JS, Oliffe JL, Dhillon HM. Engaging Men in Psychological Treatment: A Scoping Review. Am J Mens Health. 2018 Nov;12(6):1882-1900. doi: 10.1177/1557988318792157. Epub 2018 Aug 13. PMID: 30103643; PMCID: PMC6199457. https://www.ncbi.nlm.nih.gov/pmc/articles/PMC6199457/

Shafiee G, Keshtkar A, Soltani A, Ahadi Z, Larijani B, Heshmat R. Prevalence of sarcopenia in the world: a systematic review and meta- analysis of general population studies. J Diabetes Metab Disord. 2017 May 16;16:21. doi: 10.1186/s40200-017-0302-x. PMID: 28523252; PMCID: PMC5434551. https://www.ncbi.nlm.nih.gov/pmc/articles/PMC5434551/

Sher L. High and low testosterone levels may be associated with suicidal behavior in young and older men, respectively. Australian & New Zealand Journal of Psychiatry. 2013;47(5):492-493. doi:10.1177/0004867412463976. https://journals.sagepub.com/doi/10.1177/0004867412463976

Šimunić-Briški N, Dukarić V, Očić M, Madžar T, Vinicki M, Frkatović-Hodžić A, Knjaz D, Lauc G. Regular moderate physical exercise decreases Glycan Age index of biological age and reduces inflammatory potential of Immunoglobulin G. Glycoconj J. 2024 Feb;41(1):67-76. doi: 10.1007/s10719-023-10144-5. Epub 2023 Dec 26. Erratum in: Glycoconj J. 2024 Feb;41(1):77-78. doi: 10.1007/s10719-024-10146-x. PMID: 38147152; PMCID: PMC10957704. https://www.ncbi.nlm.nih.gov/pmc/articles/PMC10957704/

Slavin J. Fiber and prebiotics: mechanisms and health benefits. Nutrients. 2013 Apr 22;5(4):1417-35. doi: 10.3390/nu5041417. PMID: 23609775; PMCID: PMC3705355. https://www.ncbi.nlm.nih.gov/pmc/articles/PMC3705355/

Sleep Foundation, Is Eating Before Bed Bad? 2024. https://www.sleepfoundation.org/nutrition/is-it-bad-to-eat-before-bed#:~:text=Eating%20too%20much%20close%20to,it%20takes%20to%20fall%20asleep

Stanworth RD, Jones TH. Testosterone for the aging male; current evidence and recommended practice. Clin Interv Aging. 2008;3(1):25-44. doi: 10.2147/cia.s190. PMID: 18488876; PMCID: PMC2544367. https://www.ncbi.nlm.nih.gov/pmc/articles/PMC2544367/

Stone DM, Simon TR, Fowler KA, et al. Vital Signs: Trends in State Suicide Rates — United States, 1999–2016 and Circumstances Contributing to Suicide — 27 States, 2015. MMWR Morb Mortal Wkly Rep 2018;67:617–624. http://dx.doi.org/10.15585/mmwr.mm6722a1

Stronger By Science, Chrononutrition: Why Meal Timing, Calorie Distribution & Feeding Windows Really Do Matter. 2023. https://www.strongerbyscience.com/chrononutrition/

Susanne Knowles, Susanne Knowles, Benefits of Coaching, Positive Psychology Coaching, 10.1007/978-3-030-88995-1_5, (67-77), (2022).

Susanne Knowles, Susanne Knowles, Coaching, Positive Psychology Coaching, 10.1007/978-3-030-88995-1_4, (45-66), (2022).

T. H. Jones. Trends in Endocrinology & Metabolism, Testosterone deficiency: a risk factor for cardiovascular disease? Volume 21, Issue 8p496-503August 2010.
https://www.cell.com/trends/endocrinology-metabolism/abstract/S1043-2760(10)00048-2?_returnURL=https%3A%2F%2Flinkinghub.elsevier.com%2Fretrieve%2Fpii%2FS1043276010000482%3Fshowall%3Dtrue

T.H. Jones, Testosterone deficiency: a risk factor for cardiovascular disease? Trends In Endocrinology & Metabolism, Volume 21, Issue 8, P496-502, August 2010.
https://www.cell.com/trends/endocrinology-metabolism/abstract/S1043-2760(10)00048-2?_returnURL=https%3A%2F%2Flinkinghub.elsevier.com%2Fretrieve%2Fpii%2FS1043276010000482%3Fshowall%3Dtrue

Tactics 30 Disheartening Statistics on Mental Health Stigma. 2021.
https://etactics.com/blog/statistics-on-mental-health-stigma

Thomas G. Travison, Andre B. Araujo, Amy B. O'Donnell, Varant Kupelian, John B. McKinlay, A Population-Level Decline in Serum Testosterone Levels in American Men, The Journal of Clinical Endocrinology & Metabolism, Volume 92, Issue 1, January 2007, Pages 196–202. https://academic.oup.com/jcem/article/92/1/196/2598434?

Top Doctors, Sarcopenia. 2023. https://www.topdoctors.co.uk/medical-dictionary/sarcopenia

Travison TG, Araujo AB, Kupelian V, O'Donnell AB, McKinlay JB. The relative contributions of aging, health, and lifestyle factors to serum testosterone decline in men. J Clin Endocrinol Metab. 2007 Feb;92(2):549-55. doi: 10.1210/jc.2006-1859. Epub 2006 Dec 5. PMID: 17148559. https://pubmed.ncbi.nlm.nih.gov/17148559/

Uther M, Cleveland M, Jones R. Email Overload? Brain and Behavioral Responses to Common Messaging Alerts Are Heightened for Email Alerts and Are Associated With Job Involvement. Front Psychol. 2018 Jul 31;9:1206. doi: 10.3389/fpsyg.2018.01206. PMID: 30108531; PMCID: PMC6079232.
https://www.ncbi.nlm.nih.gov/pmc/articles/PMC6079232/

Vaamonde D, Da Silva-Grigoletto ME, García-Manso JM, Barrera N, Vaamonde-Lemos R. Physically active men show better semen parameters and hormone values than sedentary men. Eur J Appl Physiol. 2012 Sep;112(9):3267-73. doi: 10.1007/s00421-011-2304-6. Epub 2012 Jan 11. PMID: 22234399. https://pubmed.ncbi.nlm.nih.gov/22234399/

Vermeulen A, Kaufman JM, Goemaere S, van Pottelberg I. Estradiol in elderly men. Aging Male. 2002 Jun;5(2):98-102. PMID: 12198740. https://pubmed.ncbi.nlm.nih.gov/12198740/

Villablanca PA, Alegria JR, Mookadam F, Holmes DR Jr, Wright RS, Levine JA. Nonexercise activity thermogenesis in obesity management. Mayo Clin Proc. 2015 Apr;90(4):509-19. doi: 10.1016/j.mayocp.2015.02.001. PMID: 25841254.
https://www.ncbi.nlm.nih.gov/pubmed/25841254

# REFERENCES

Walker ER, McGee RE, Druss BG. Mortality in mental disorders and global disease burden implications: a systematic review and meta-analysis. JAMA Psychiatry. 2015 Apr;72(4):334-41. doi: 10.1001/jamapsychiatry.2014.2502. Erratum in: JAMA Psychiatry. 2015 Jul;72(7):736. doi: 10.1001/jamapsychiatry.2015.0937. Erratum in: JAMA Psychiatry. 2015 Dec;72(12):1259. doi: 10.1001/jamapsychiatry.2015.2246. PMID: 25671328; PMCID: PMC4461039.
https://pubmed.ncbi.nlm.nih.gov/25671328/

Weber KS, Setchell KD, Stocco DM, Lephart ED. Dietary soy-phytoestrogens decrease testosterone levels and prostate weight without altering LH, prostate 5alpha-reductase or testicular steroidogenic acute regulatory peptide levels in adult male Sprague-Dawley rats. J Endocrinol. 2001 Sep;170(3):591-9. doi: 10.1677/joe.0.1700591. PMID: 11524239.
https://pubmed.ncbi.nlm.nih.gov/11524239/

Wong, Y. J., Owen, J., Gabana, N. T., Brown, J. W., McInnis, S., Toth, P., & Gilman, L. (2016). Does gratitude writing improve the mental health of psychotherapy clients? Evidence from a randomized controlled trial. Psychotherapy Research, 28(2), 192–202. https://doi.org/10.1080/10503307.2016.1169332.
https://www.tandfonline.com/doi/citedby/10.1080/10503307.2016.1169332?scroll=top&needAccess=true

World Cancer Research Fund, Prostate Cancer, 2014.
https://www.wcrf-uk.org/cancer-types/prostate-cancer/?gad_source=1&gclid=CjOKCQjwpP63BhDYARIsAOQkATY-hKG5CSa4K4tv9RcTNJEW7PrDALXHydxwF6d8a5gQGDFKbqljYQO8aAgWBEALw_wcB

World Health Organisation, Depressive Disorder. 2023. https://www.who.int/news-room/fact-sheets/detail/depression

World Health Organisation, Mental Health of Older Adults, 2023.
https://www.who.int/news-room/fact-sheets/detail/mental-health-of-older-adults

Wu H, Flint AJ, Qi Q, van Dam RM, Sampson LA, Rimm EB, Holmes MD, Willett WC, Hu FB, Sun Q. Association between dietary whole grain intake and risk of mortality: two large prospective studies in US men and women. JAMA Intern Med. 2015 Mar;175(3):373-84. doi: 10.1001/jamainternmed.2014.6283. PMID: 25559238; PMCID: PMC4429593.
https://pubmed.ncbi.nlm.nih.gov/25559238/

Yaribeygi H, Panahi Y, Sahraei H, Johnston TP, Sahebkar A. The impact of stress on body function: A review. EXCLI J. 2017 Jul 21;16:1057-1072. doi: 10.17179/excli2017-480. PMID: 28900385; PMCID: PMC5579396.
https://www.ncbi.nlm.nih.gov/pmc/articles/PMC5579396/

Yeomans MR. Alcohol, appetite and energy balance: is alcohol intake a risk factor for obesity? Physiol Behav. 2010 Apr 26;100(1):82-9. doi: 10.1016/j.physbeh.2010.01.012. Epub 2010 Jan 22. PMID: 20096714.
https://pubmed.ncbi.nlm.nih.gov/20096714/

YouGov, How Often Brits Exercise. 2024.
https://yougov.co.uk/topics/society/trackers/how-often-brits-exercise?period=1yr&crossBreak=female

Young SN. How to increase serotonin in the human brain without drugs. J Psychiatry Neurosci. 2007 Nov;32(6):394-9. PMID: 18043762; PMCID: PMC2077351. https://www.ncbi.nlm.nih.gov/pmc/articles/PMC2077351/

Yousafzai, Aziz ur Rehman et al. "SERUM TESTOSTERONE LEVELS IN YOUNG MALE PATIENTS WITH MAJOR DEPRESSION." Journal of Ayub Medical College Abbottabad 12 (2000).
https://www.semanticscholar.org/paper/SERUM-TESTOSTERONE-LEVELS-IN-YOUNG-MALE-PATIENTS-Yousafzai-Yousuf/eedad422dda6b774ea2d93915c3b40fabcd7ae22

Zhang M, Jia J, Yang Y, Zhang L, Wang X. Effects of exercise interventions on cognitive functions in healthy populations: A systematic review and meta-analysis. Ageing Res Rev. 2023 Dec;92:102116. doi: 10.1016/j.arr.2023.102116. Epub 2023 Nov 3. PMID: 37924980. https://pubmed.ncbi.nlm.nih.gov/37924980/

Zueger R, Annen H, Ehlert U. Testosterone and cortisol responses to acute and prolonged stress during officer training school. Stress. 2023 Jan;26(1):2199886. doi: 10.1080/10253890.2023.2199886. PMID: 37014073. https://pubmed.ncbi.nlm.nih.gov/37014073/